Moving Stretch

Moving Stretch

Work Your Fascia to Free Your Body

Suzanne Wylde

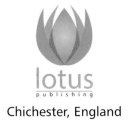

Chichester, England

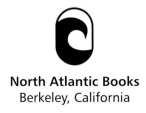

North Atlantic Books
Berkeley, California

First published in 2017 by
Lotus Publishing
Apple Tree Cottage, Inlands Road, Nutbourne, Chichester, PO18 8RJ and
North Atlantic Books
Berkeley, California

Disclaimer

The stretches are for healthy, physically able people. If you are currently ill, injured, pregnant or have any health or physical limitations then you should check with your doctor or healthcare provider before starting to stretch. None of the advice in this book is a substitute for medical advice. The reader should regularly consult a physician in matters relating to his/her health and particularly with respect to any symptoms that may require diagnosis or medical attention. When you undertake these stretches it is at your sole discretion and risk.

The information in this book is meant to supplement, not replace, proper stretching education. Like any physical activity, stretching poses some inherent risk. The author and publisher advise readers to take full responsibility for their safety and know their limits. Before practicing the techniques described in this book, be sure that you are in a safe area, and do not take risks beyond your level of experience, physical ability, and comfort level.

Photographs Lucy Arrowsmith, www.lucy-arrowsmith.com
Cover Photograph Karen Yeomans, www.karenyeomans.com
Text and Cover Design Wendy Craig
Printed and Bound in Malaysia by Tien Wah Press

Moving Stretch: Work Your Fascia to Free Your Body is sponsored by the Society for the Study of Native Arts and Sciences, a nonprofit educational corporation whose goals are to develop an educational and crosscultural perspective linking various scientific, social, and artistic fields; to nurture a holistic view of arts, sciences, humanities, and healing; and to publish and distribute literature on the relationship of mind, body, and nature.

British Library Cataloguing-in-Publication Data
A CIP record for this book is available from the British Library
ISBN 978 1 905367 74 0 (Lotus Publishing)
ISBN 978 1 62317 175 9 (North Atlantic Books)

Library of Congress Cataloging-in-Publication Data
Names: Wylde, Suzanne, author.
Title: Moving stretch : move your fascia to free your body / Suzanne Wylde.
Description: Berkeley, California : North Atlantic Books, 2017. | Includes bibliographical references and index.
Identifiers: LCCN 2016056337 (print) | LCCN 2017008875 (ebook) | ISBN 9781623171759 (paperback) | ISBN 9781623171766 (ebook)
Subjects: LCSH: Stretching exercises. | Fasciae (Anatomy) | BISAC: HEALTH & FITNESS / Exercise. | MEDICAL / Alternative Medicine. | SPORTS & RECREATION / Training.
Classification: LCC RA781.63 .W95 2017 (print) | LCC RA781.63 (ebook) | DDC 613.7/182—dc23
LC record available at https://lccn.loc.gov/2016056337

For Nathan, Emily, Danny, James and the little Cakes.

You already know that anything is possible. Thank you for inspiring me every day.

Contents

Acknowledgments

I want to thank my clients and students for letting me try things out with them, using the stretches and inspiring me with their progress; without you guys there would be no *Moving Stretch*. I also want to thank my editor, Jon, who waited very patiently for the manuscript and helped me with lots of random questions and also Hannah for the extra guidance!

Sweaty Betty generously provided the clothes for all of the female models in this book and Simon and Fleur were especially helpful in getting the gorgeous outfits to me safely and on time. I think their mission of helping to inspire women to become fit and empowered is amazing, and one very close to my heart. And thank you to the ladies who came to stretch and be photographed! Nikki was one of the main models, very kindly giving her time and energy, as well as her focus as she demonstrated lots and lots of stretches. Natalia Hinds came and made the cover amazing with her sparkly presence and also helped to liven up the beginning chapters of the book; I'm glad we met by chance and that you happened to be an actress and also perfect for my front cover! A big, big thank you also to Katie, Daria, Amelia, and Carly. You guys posed like the superstars you are and stretched every day for a month. I have to say you were all looking even more fabulous afterwards!

2XU were epic as I reached out to them at short notice, and Aidan and Mike managed to race against the clock and get me clothes for the men in this book. They make such high-quality technical gear, the guys were really happy to have it for their exercise outside of their stretching also.

To the men; thank you for overcoming any natural camera-shyness. You all looked amazing! Especially after the month of stretching you undertook. Brad was very enthusiastic in giving his time and focus in demonstrating the stretches as the other main model of the book. Javier and Avi, I want to thank you both for your dedication in stretching every day for a month. I am so glad that you got some good changes!

The people who made the book as good-looking as it is are two wonderful photographers. I want to thank Lucy Arrowsmith, who took all of the photos inside the book; you are a great support and source of inspiration (and attention to detail, stick that mat down!). Also Karen Yeomans, who made the cover photo better even than in my imagination, thank you for your creativity and your tenacity in getting the right shot; I think it's beautiful.

I'd like to thank Tom Myers and Julian Baker for allowing me to interview them. Tom, as the creator of Anatomy Trains, is a guiding light on all things fascia and I was very lucky to have the chance to ask him some questions to clarify what I thought about fascia and stretching, especially as he has 40 years of experience! Julian Baker is a leading Bowen practitioner and expert in fascia matters and I was fascinated by his unique approach to bodywork and very grateful to have been able to attend a dissection with him for the purpose of looking at the anatomy of the fascia within the body. Even though I am not the most academic person or best versed in fascia research, they were both very patient with my open-ended questions, so thank you.

I would like to say thank you to Simon Mawer for recommending a malacologist when I was trying to find out if slugs have fascia and to Professor Gonzalo Giribet who managed to answer this slippery question (I would also like to thank all the friends I kept boring with the fact that slugs have around 27,000 teeth!). I would also like to thank Simon Connor from the Museo Egizio in Turin for allowing me to use a photo of their Egyptian dancer, as well as the many other people who gave me permission to reproduce their photographs. Thank you also to Charles, who I met at a NYE party in the woods and who thought my ideas had potential and gave me a lot of great advice. PR Whizz Georgie Wolfinden at Blossom Consulting has been wonderful at helping me to spread the word, huge thanks Georgie!

On a more personal note, I would like to thank my Mum and Dad, Simon and Jen, and my whole family for being supportive when I needed it most. I'd like to thank my friends for remaining friends through fairly lengthy periods of writing-reclusiveness and for offering all kinds of help. A book definitely doesn't write itself—but an author doesn't write it by herself either. Not a stretching book anyway! Thanks to Graeme Waterworth for introducing me to resistance stretching and encouraging me in my work. I also want to say a big thank you to Raj Nandrup, my first Tai Chi teacher who set me on this whole crazy path and for being his own special brand of lovely. And thank you to Lily Lai for using her PhD super-brain to cross-examine me. I would also like to say a special thank you to Jonathan and the staff at Triyoga, who have given me so much support and guidance as I have emerged from my treatment room more and more to do things in the bright light of the wider world.

A special thank you to Mark Gratton for the impersonations, walks and adventures that took my mind off the book when I needed it as well as tons of moral support. I couldn't have done it without you. I'd also like to thank one of my oldest friends for her support through rain or shine (and in Britain that's mostly the former) Suzette you have the rare ability to eat hot sauce at any time of day.

And to all the people who read this book and stretch along to it, thank you for using what I have made so that it has value. That is what it is all about in the end; sharing information that hopefully empowers people and makes them a little stronger, freer and happier. Thank you all!

Suzanne Wylde

Preface

Day after day I see people on the streets, hunched over, lopsided, moving with difficulty, tense, in pain, needlessly "less than." Less than they could be if only their bodies were free to be strong, upright, confident, able to move without restriction. It makes me feel a bit sad and a bit frustrated sometimes, because in most cases, everything that people need in order to have strong, upright bodies is already all there. Most people just do not know how to get rid of the limitations caused by their lifestyles and movement patterns. This limitation and restriction can even affect active people, whose posture, performance, and alignment suffer as a result. Over time these limitations often lead to injury, worsening posture, and, in my opinion, premature aging.

If large numbers of people are walking around with a burden that they could cast off with just a little regular effort, wouldn't it make sense for them to do so? And tight fascia that holds you down and bent out of shape is just that: an unnecessary burden. I am not so naïve that I expect everyone with poor posture and pain to pick this book up and start stretching. But if a few do, if you start to have a better life, with more movement, more freedom in your body, better performance in sport, and maybe even more enjoyment in physical movement as a whole, then I will be happy.

My work up until now has been to help people feel better, and often wonderful, one at a time. The results my clients get have often been amazing and satisfying to them and to me, with transformations that lead their friends to ask what they are doing differently. However, up until now it has been limited to a one-on-one, or small group class basis. Now I hope to be able to help greater numbers of people to feel better in their own bodies, through the techniques I have set out in this book.

And it is not just yourself that will be affected by your stretching practice. Through being freer and more open physically you will inspire and encourage those around you to be better than they already are. So, if you have difficulty in motivating yourself to improve your body for yourself, think of your partners and spouses, your children and parents, your friends and business colleagues and imagine everyone being just that little bit stronger and healthier. Don't you want your friends and family to stay moving, strong, and healthy for as long as possible?

As we learn and develop in skill and experience, different teachers, movers, authors, speakers and bodyworkers come forward to offer their own unique piece of the puzzle of how to be fit, tall, strong, functional, free to move, and happy. I hope that the piece I am offering is useful and gives you a practical way to use resistance stretching to improve your body and your life.

To everyone who wants to have a happier, freer, stronger, and more upright and naturally flexible body, I wrote this book for you.

Introduction

Welcome to this book on stretching your fascia. I am excited for you because you still do not know how much resistance stretching can benefit you, but I do! I have seen the impressed, surprised, and happy expressions on the faces of my clients for several years now as they become more open, taller, faster, more graceful, more powerful and flexible in quite a short space of time.

I am so happy to have this opportunity to give you all the information you need to do this for yourself and improve under your own steam, as I only have the capacity to stretch around 20 people a week and teach a small class of around five. I love working with my clients, but 25 a week is not exactly a revolution in world health, if you see what I'm saying. But now, armed with all the information you need, you can create amazing changes at home and at your own pace for only the price of this book. I think that's pretty great.

You probably picked up this book (or opened it electronically) because you need something to change. Whether it is your hamstrings, your height, or that you are hurting, you need a physical improvement, and you want it sooner rather than later. So let's jump in with some of the most common questions about stretching the fascia with resistance and how you can get started.

Resistance Stretching Is …

A form of stretching with two key elements, resistance and movement. The resistance comes from tensing your muscles and the movement from moving your limbs or torso (or both) in a certain way for each stretch, whilst maintaining that tension. You resist in order to engage the fascia and then you move in order to recondition and stretch the fascia. Resistance stretching was created by Bob Cooley, who I originally trained with in Boston and gives great results in both strength and flexibility and unlike other stretching techniques, can even re-shape your body if needed.

What Resistance Stretching Is Not

Although it contains the word *resistance*, it does not utilize resistance bands (the stretchy bands used for strength training) and it is not a dedicated form of resistance training per se (although it does strengthen you). It is not at all like Pilates, although some movements do involve a lot of core as a side benefit. It is unlike yoga in that it is mostly about moving through your own resistance, rather than moving between, and holding certain poses. It is not really about poses at all, but movements. It is not overly formal; you can do a set routine, make your own routine, or do a couple of stretches only. If you attend self-stretching classes in resistance stretching (a Moving Stretch® class anyway) no two classes will be the same. It is also unlike many other forms of stretching which focus more on individual muscles and the end of the range of motion.

What Moving Stretch® Is

You have probably only just heard of resistance stretching, so hopefully I will not confuse you too much when I say that there are also different kinds of resistance stretching. The stretches, routines, and technique in this book are from my method named Moving Stretch® (so named because all of the stretches involve movement of some kind). I created it because I saw a need for a simple, accessible, easy-to-learn-and-use system of resistance stretching. Moving Stretches powerfully affect the fascia to release and transform your body. They are also pretty fun and engaging, I hope you enjoy them!

What Fascia Is

Fascia is a type of connective tissue that runs from our head to our feet and connects every part of us. It makes us the shape that we are, holding us together and everything in place. Initially thought to be not very interesting at all, it now is of great interest and even has its own books, studies, and conferences, all of which should let you know that it is now of great import (it really has been all along!). When you want to improve the structure of your body, working on the tissue that gives it its structure is a very sensible thing to do.

How I Came to Write This Book

Once upon a time there was a 15-year-old girl who could not touch her toes or sit cross-legged without feeling intense pain in her hips. She could run with a larger teenager on her back but she was about as likely to do the splits as she was to become the president of Russia. In fact, the latter may have been more likely. Now, double that age, she is writing this book (yes, as you already guessed, that teen is me) about flexibility and the fascia. I still cannot do the splits, but I have a functional body that can sit, walk, bend, jump, and move in most ways without limitation or pain, is nicely in balance, and feels naturally strong and flexible in all the ways I need and want to be.

So many people walk in through my door, inflexible, stiff, bent over, out of balance, and out of alignment, who have never really understood how to stretch in a way that is effective and satisfying for them. Having been in that condition myself, I know very well what it feels like to have a body that feels intractable, plank-like, unyielding, embarrassing in yoga classes. I never understood how the others gently folded themselves in half or curled themselves elegantly, bodies of plasticine and minds as one, while my cheeks reddened with effort as I struggled, my defiant toddler of a body refusing flatly to comply.

When I discovered stretching with resistance I experienced immediate benefits in my posture and a delicious freedom of movement in my body. Resistance stretching works on the fascia as well as the muscles; not only to increase flexibility, but to recondition the body. In a way it is like bodywork that you do to yourself, but with more lasting changes. And so when I started stretching I found myself changing, developing a more resilient body with a greater, yet sustainable and healthy, range of movement.

The great thing is that, aside from increases in flexibility, there are some serious strength benefits. This means that if you are naturally flexible but not very strong, resistance stretching will give you the strength that you need to boost your stability. And if you are already generally strong, you will also strengthen yourself in the areas where you are weak (most of which you will not realize are weak until you try to use them).

I have watched my clients improve so much and now, after years of practice and experience as a trainer and having created this particular technique, I hope to be able to help many more people through this book. I sincerely hope that it becomes dog-eared, scribbled-on, thumbed-through, wrinkled, and happily battered through frequent use and re-reading and that it helps you and yours to feel better. By using these stretches, you should feel lighter, stronger and more flexible, graceful, upright and empowered.

How to Use this Book

I know you must be excited by now, but before you dive into your first stretches, please take a look at the How to Stretch section (Chapter 9) to make sure you are doing the exercises in a safe and effective way. There is a little more to stretching, especially resistance stretching, than meets the eye and if you do the stretches incorrectly you may lose out on the benefit or even accidentally strain yourself, so it is important that you get your head around the technique first. Through my teaching practice I have learned specifically what questions beginners tend to ask and which errors are common, so I have also included this information in the How to Stretch section.

Before you start stretching, I recommend that you do an initial Flexibility Assessment (Chapter 8), as this will show you where you need to do the most work and will also be a great way to measure your improvement as you progress in your stretching practice. You can then start to work through the individual stretches for the different areas of the body in the Moving Stretches section (Chapter 10). I suggest that you take your time to familiarize yourself with the instructions and the movements and work through the stretches at your own pace. After doing some of the individual stretches, you can go to the Moving Stretch Routines (Chapter 11) to try a specific stretching plan.

The most crucial thing to master in order to get the most out of your stretching is how to create continuous and steady tension in your muscles throughout the movement. This tension engages the fascia and ensures that it is being stretched alongside your muscles and other tissues. The How to Stretch section (Chapter 9) shows you how to do this effectively to get the best results.

The About Stretching section (Chapter 1) gives you some background information on stretching and flexibility. The About Fascia section (Chapter 2) is designed to give you the background information you need in order to understand what your fascia is, why it matters to you, and how you can work with it in order to have a healthier, more flexible body. If you are interested, then the Resistance Stretching and Fascia section (Chapter 3) will give you the basics of how resistance stretching the fascia works and A New Look at Stretching and Flexibility (Chapter 4) discusses what being flexible means, and how a regular stretching practice may be able to change you. We also cover Why Some People Aren't Stretchy (And Others Are) (Chapter 5), some of the main Benefits of Stretching (Chapter 6), some information on the Best Attitude for Stretching (Chapter 12), as well as some extra Motivation for Stretching (Chapter 13).

To keep it accessible the book is divided into short, readable sections, (in case you are busy or have a short attention span) (just kidding—mostly—thanks smartphones!). If you are confused about any particular points there is also an FAQ section with all the most commonly asked questions (Chapter 7). You do not have to read the whole book from cover to cover, but please do remember to read the How to Stretch section before you begin stretching.

Resistance stretching and fascia are both pretty new to the table, so there is not always as much research as we would like, particularly regarding resistance stretching. I have supported most of the factual points in this book with information from studies and experts, but a lot of what I have written comes from my hands-on practice and is what I believe to be true. I rely mostly on results; for example the before and after photos in the Stretching Routines section show the effect of resistance stretching for 10–20 minutes every day for 30 days. However, maintaining its flexibility, my system will continue to grow and evolve, updating its technique and learning from the most current research in order to serve people in the best way possible.

From a hardened shell to a happy moveable creature, resistance stretching has set me free. I hope it does the same for you, empowering you, opening up your sphere of movement and influence and letting you feel tall, strong, and happy. I hope that you get amazing results from your stretching!

1 About Stretching

It is interesting that something so natural and essential to our well-being as stretching is still at times as poorly understood, controversial or out of reach for many. Because stretching has principally been regarded as a side dish to other physical activities and therapies such as dance, exercise, physiotherapy, martial arts, and others, it is rarely presented as a whole meal. Therefore our knowledge of stretching and how to do it is often incomplete, with different groups of people possessing specialized information relevant to what they themselves are doing, but no one having the whole picture.

Resistance stretching is quite niche, but it is fairly easy to pick up, very adaptable to each individual, and fits in very well with other bodywork modalities. As such, I think it is a great choice to get stuck into as your primary method of stretching and taking care of your body. However, before I tell you all about resistance stretching and how to do it, let us have a look at how this whole business of stretching started.

The History of Stretching

Ever since creatures have had musculoskeletal (as well as fascial) systems, stretching has existed to maintain them. The impulse to stretch is just as innate, instinctive, and vital to our health as breathing, eating, and drinking water. Animals, and cats especially, stay supple in such an effortless way; a day never passes without them fluidly pushing themselves into and through a whole-body tensioned and yawning stretch. This type of stretching is known as *pandiculation*, which is a type of resistance stretching.

We do this too; when we first wake up we strongly tense our muscles and then push through that into a satisfyingly strong and opening stretch. Staying supple and able to react with smooth, fast, and powerful movements made us successful at finding food and losing predators, thus ensuring our survival. Now that survival for many of us is secured through our ability to carry out tasks using our brains instead of brawn, our physicality has been sidelined. But more than that, our stationary (and a little unnatural) positions at desks have caused many of us to be hunched, tight, low on energy, and weaker than we could be. Even if you have a job that means you are on your feet all day, absent-minded hunching over smartphones, tablets, laptops, and on sofas may be undermining your posture and your physical power more than you realize.

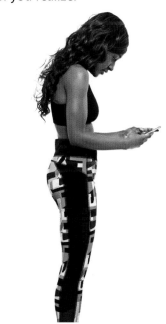

Figure 1.1 Poor posture.

But even before smart phone use and sedentary lifestyles made stretching a very good idea, it had already been widely practiced throughout a multitude of cultures and in different eras. Stretching as a system of specific movements and exercises has its origins in many ancient civilizations, including the yoga of the East and the physical disciplines of Ancient Greece. It is clear that humans have seen the benefit of a deliberate and targeted stretching practice in terms of health, performance, and alleviating pain and injury for a very long time.

The first recorded mention of yoga was in the Rig Veda ("knowledge of praise") 3,000 years ago. It was, and is, a method of personal development that works on the mind, body, and spirit through mental and physical practices, but its original purpose was purely for spiritual development. This may not always translate across to yoga practice in the West, partly because it goes much deeper than some people want to go or take the time to explore. However, there are many very accomplished yoga teachers in the West and in general the ones I am privileged to know have great bodies (balanced and in a good "state") as well as a calm and open disposition. This quote shows the importance of the mind–body connection in yoga:

> *"You cannot do yoga. Yoga is your natural state. What you can do are yoga exercises, which may reveal to you where you are resisting your natural state."*
>
> *Sharon Gannon*

This is quite a contrast from standing in PE with your teacher telling you to bend at the waist and reach for your plimsolls! In fact the origins of stretching in the West are, like the foundations of Western medicine, to be found in the lifestyle and health philosophy of Ancient Greece. Athletics, gymnastics, wrestling and running were the staple exercises of the time and the pioneering coaches were none other than **Hippocrates, Aristotle, and Plato**. The mind–body connection was extremely important, but more in the light of optimal physical health

and fitness forming the basis of a good mind, rather than working on the body in a specific way to achieve spiritual development. Athletes would get a massage and stretch after each training session as part of their recovery procedure and it is interesting to note that while our technology, society, and day-to-day lives have changed so much since the time of Hippocrates, our bodies have not, and therefore require a similar kind of care. There are not many details of the exact stretches that were popular in Ancient Greece, but it is known that they used stretching to enhance their exercise, dancing, health, military training, and therapeutic work.[1]

There is even evidence that stretching was an important aspect of physical training in Ancient Egypt over 4,000 years ago.

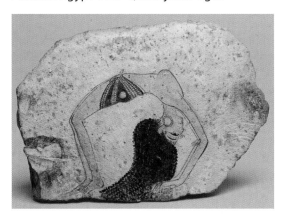

Figure 1.2 Example from Ancient Egypt of the full bridge exercise that is still performed today. Egyptian dancer © Museo Egizio.

So if the history of stretching is so long, why has it developed so little compared to other exercise and strengthening techniques? I believe that this is in part due to the fact that most people believe that the fairly simple and linear "normal" (properly known as static) stretches they were taught in school are "as good as it gets," (which is very far from the pandiculation of animals or resistance stretching you will learn in this book). Other, newer techniques are usually known only to therapists or physiotherapists and their clients. However, this information rarely filters through to the general public. Therefore even when there are developments in stretching, most people sadly do not have access to them.

1 Porcari et al., 2015.

A Little Bit about the Theory of Stretching

The science around stretching usually focuses on the physiology of muscles, but as resistance stretching focuses on affecting the fascia, we will have a quick look at both.

The physiology of the body whilst stretching, especially that of the muscles, is pretty firmly established (although much about the fascia's response to stretching remains to be studied). The type of muscles we are concerned with are skeletal muscles as they are the ones that we stretch. They are attached to bones by tendons and move the body by pulling on the bones. They are made of bundles of muscle fibers, which can contract and relax. The muscles and even individual muscle fibers are wrapped in fascia.

There are three main types of muscle contraction:

- **Isometric**—a contraction without movement (i.e., when you push against something that does not move)

- **Concentric**—when you contract your muscle and it shortens (e.g., when lifting a weight)

- **Eccentric**—when your muscle gets longer while it is tense and resisting that lengthening movement (lowering a weight slowly, for example, or resistance stretching)

When a muscle is stretched it has a little internal monitor inside it, called the muscle spindle, that records how much it is lengthening. The muscle spindle lives right in the belly of your muscle and can trigger the *stretch reflex*, which is an involuntary contraction in a muscle that is getting longer; the longer it gets, the more it contracts. This is to safeguard the muscle from overstretching.

It is a little bit like sending an accountant along with a shopaholic on a shopping trip, just to be on the safe side. The theory is that if you want to be able to stretch further, you should let your muscle spindle get used to the muscles being longer so that it does not counteract your stretch. This is one aspect of the huge neurological aspect of stretching (it is not all about muscles and fascia, the nervous system is very involved too).

The counterpart to the muscle spindle is the Golgi tendon organ, which lives between the muscle and the tendon. Its job is to notice how much the muscle is contracting and it can override the contraction and force the muscle to relax instead. Like the muscle spindle it is protective, but in the other direction. It is a bit like the valve on a pressure cooker, protecting the muscles from force that could harm them.

When Fascia Stretches

Less is known about how the fascia behaves during stretching than about muscles, as it has not been researched as extensively (although some people classify ligaments as part of the fascial system because they are made of very similar stuff, and therefore feel that research into ligaments can give us an insight into the nature of fascia). We do know that the fascia is affected by stretching differently to muscles because it has a different architecture and a different MO. Some of the main functions of fascia are to provide structure in our bodies, to offer back-up strength to our muscles and also power through elastic recoil. It can contract, but not like a muscle does, and it also stretches differently.

The phrase "muscles are elastic and fascia is plastic" describes the fact that muscles can stretch and elongate, then spring back into shape, but that fascia can only stretch if it is stretched slowly, when it deforms, but if stretched too quickly it may tear, causing pain and dysfunction. Tom Myers, who is one of the foremost fascia experts, says the best way to demonstrate this is with a plastic bag (or plastic wrap as pictured here) being pulled apart slowly and stretching versus being pulled apart quickly and tearing.

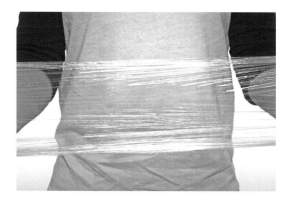

Figure 1.3A Fascia being stretched slowly.

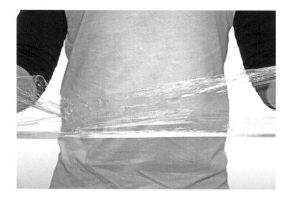

Figure 1.3B Fascia being stretched too fast and tearing.

Our goal when stretching is not simply to make the fascia "longer" and stretch as hard as we can. This is often not even desirable, especially in people who are naturally flexible, or some specific areas of the body, that require stability more than increased range of motion.

Because it is the tensioned part of a tensegral structure (a combination of the words "tension" and "integrity;" for more information see the next chapter) it can move in any direction, naturally resist movement of any kind, distribute force all throughout the fascial system, spring back into shape (as long as you do not pull it too far) and also the whole system is affected by a change in one part of the whole.[2] These amazing features mean that when you stretch fascia, you stretch the *whole* of your fascia. That is quite

a leap away from the more reductionist view of seeing the body as a collection of separate moving parts that you can only affect one at a time.

Our fascia is not always well laid-out and organized; it can also become a bit messy. Fascial adhesions, which are bits of our fascia that have become stuck together internally, are not only found in the bodies of those who have suffered severe trauma to the body, such as a motorbike accident; in fact most of us have some adhesions in our fascia. They are caused by abnormal physical strain, which can even result from poor posture and physical habits. Once we have them, they can grow in size and can have knock-on effects such as restricting movement and causing pain. The great thing about resistance stretching the fascia is that it can "clean the fascia up." When the fascia is stretched, any disorganized fibers in it are reorganized in line with the direction of the tension[3] and this allows adhesions and scar tissue to be rehabilitated through stretching.

According to Tom Myers, resistance stretching the fascia may affect the hyaluronic acid (a viscous, slippery substance in the fascia) beneficially by breaking down long sticky chains into shorter ones. This increases the lubrication and "gliding" within the tissue.[4] I believe this could be one of the ways that resistance stretching increases ease and gracefulness of movement as well as improving dexterity.

Resistance stretching also has an impact on the body as a whole, affecting all the holistic "nets"—the neural, the circulatory, and the fibrous. This means that stretching with resistance may benefit the body in ways that go beyond simple increases in range of motion.

Now that you know some more about how fascia stretches, hopefully you will understand why we will focus on reconditioning, spring cleaning, and working our fascia out, rather than trying to make it looser.

2 Avison, 2015.
3 Appleton, 2010.
4 Myers, 2016.

The Many Kinds of Stretching

Before we look at resistance stretching, let us take a few minutes to look at other methods of stretching, as set out in Table 1.1, so that you understand the ways that resistance stretching is similar to, and distinct from, them.

Type of stretching	Description	How it is similar, or different to, resistance stretching?
1. Static stretching	This is the one you know, where you reach as far as you can and then try to push even further (bending over to touch your toes, for example). Static stretching focuses on increasing the range of motion through pushing beyond it, whilst keeping the muscles fairly relaxed. This is great for those who need a large range of motion such as dancers; however, it has been shown to diminish power output in athletes of explosive sports such as sprinting.	Resistance stretching focuses on moving through the whole range of motion with tension in the muscles, rather than going straight to the end of the range with relaxed muscles. This can be hard for people to learn as going straight to the end of the range and pushing is often a deeply ingrained habit. Based on my experience of working with athletes, I have not observed a reduced power output, but rather an increase in performance. I believe this is due to the smaller ROM of Moving Stretches as well as its strengthening effect. This is discussed further in the section Stretching as a Warm-up for Sport (in Chapter 9).

2. Passive or assisted stretching	This is very similar to static stretching, but either you, or another person, holds part of you in a stretched position. It feels great to have a trainer stretch you beyond your normal ranges of motion after a workout. However, be careful not to overdo it, because a study found that there was a sizeable electromechanical delay (which means it takes longer from when the muscle starts to work to the time it actually produces a movement) after passive stretching, which means people who need to move fast such as athletes do not perform as well after being stretched.[1] PNF (proprioceptive neuromuscular facilitation), which incorporates the use of tension in the muscles, had a much smaller effect on electromechanical delay in this study. It was also thought to be better for maintaining dynamic joint stability (which just means how stable your joints are when they're moving).	There is an assisted version of resistance stretching but it still involves resistance, unlike this form of stretching, where the muscles being stretched are passive. On the plus side, resistance stretching can produce very responsive and dexterous movement in people. On the downside it requires more effort than passive stretching. From my experience of working with athletes, I believe that resistance stretching is unlikely to substantially increase electromechanical delay as it incorporates muscle tension, as PNF does, and probably also maintains dynamic joint stability. As stated above, the athletes I have worked with have experienced improved, rather than reduced, performance.
3. Active stretching	You hold a position without any outside help, i.e., with your leg up in the air for around 10–15 seconds. By contracting the muscles on one side of the body you allow the muscles on the opposite side to relax and lengthen.	Resistance stretching is almost the opposite of this, as it is not static and you are contracting the muscles that you are stretching, rather than only the ones on the opposite side, while you move.
4. PNF stretching	Short for proprioceptive neuromuscular facilitation, PNF was initially developed as a method for rehabilitating stroke victims. You go to the end of the range of motion and then contract your muscle (by pushing against someone holding you in a fixed position) for around 5 seconds only, before relaxing and possibly going further in the stretch before repeating.	It is similar to resistance stretching in that you contract the muscle you are stretching, but in PNF you only do that at the end of the range of motion in a fixed position and only for a very short time. In resistance stretching you contract the muscles and move against that tension through the whole range of motion.

5. Isometric stretching	If you remember that before we mentioned that an isometric contraction is one without movement, this will give you a clue as to what this type of stretching consists of. You go to the end of the range of motion, contract your muscles for around 7–15 seconds, relax and repeat. A common example is the calf stretch at the wall, where you are pushing against the wall and not going anywhere.	This form of stretching is similar to PNF, but the contractions are held for longer. Even so, the effect is very different to resistance stretching, where the main effect comes from the combination of movement and tension combined.
6. Ballistic stretching	This is almost as dynamic as it sounds, using explosive movements to push the body into a stretched position and allowing the elastic recoil of the body to pull it back again. It consists of lots of bouncing, falling into lunges, swinging the arms rapidly and other fast movements.	Resistance stretching is much more controlled, comfortable and "safe feeling" than ballistic stretching, which for some people, may shock the body into tightening up. Because a lot of the recoil is provided by the fascia, this type of movement will not persuade it to relax and lengthen, but rather the opposite. Also, you can do resistance stretching without conditioning your body first, but this is not advisable with ballistic stretching.
7. Dynamic stretching	This also involves movement, but in a much slower and controlled manner. You never go past your natural range of movement and it seems to be more geared toward increasing mobility rather than specifically increasing the range of motion. The movements include a variety of swinging limbs, twists, and natural movements.	The slower, controlled nature of this stretching is much more similar to resistance stretching, but the actual movements are quite different and in resistance stretching we continuously tense the muscles.

8. Active isolated stretching	In this system of stretching you move into a stretch by contracting the muscles on the other side of the body (i.e., the quads, when stretching the hamstrings) and hold it for a very short amount of time. The theory is that you avoid triggering the stretch reflex by only holding it for 2 seconds, but the research does not seem to bear this out.[2]	Like resistance stretching this method involves purposefully contracting the muscles, but unlike it, it contracts the ones on the other side of the body, allowing the lengthened muscle to relax, whereas in resistance stretching we stretch the muscle that we are contracting. Also when resistance stretching we do not hold the stretch, as the stretch happens whilst we are moving.
9. Loaded stretching	When performing loaded stretching you take your muscle through its whole range whilst it simultaneously contracts. The reason that it is contracting is that there is a weight pulling it, and your limb is resisting that. So your limb and the weight are both going in the same direction, which moves you into a stretch, but your muscles have the brakes on, which means they are continuously contracted.	This is a lot like resistance stretching except that in resistance stretching you do not use weights; you either use yourself, or in the case of assisted stretching, someone else is stretching you. The advantage of resistance stretching over loaded stretching is that the force that is moving you can be continuously adjusted for the best effect and also for safety. When a weight is pulling you down it does not know if it is about to pull you too far or through a much weaker area, possibly injuring you; therefore I would say that resistance stretching is safer and more nuanced.

Table 1.1 Types of stretching.

Now that we have looked at stretching in general and the many other types of stretching, let's take a look at fascia to give you an insight into what you will be working with when you start to resistance stretch.

About Fascia

Fascia has been around since living beings have had muscles. Humans, mammals, and fish all have fascia that forms a tidy pocket for muscles and helps to keep them and other bits in the right place as well as preventing them from rubbing together while they do their thing. The shape, thickness and composition of fascia depends on its job. In fish, for example, the superficial (closer to the skin) fascia merges much more with the deeper (in the body) fascia,[5] probably because it is not very useful to fish to have "slidey" skin. Compare this to the skin of a Shar Pei and you may get an idea of how fascial structure affects anatomy (although the primary cause of the wrinkles in this breed is excess mucin rather than loose fascia, which is a result of this condition rather than the cause). Because fascia is so key to shape and function, therefore, it is clear that keeping it in good condition should be a priority for us all.

What Fascia Is, Exactly

Fascia is a type of connective tissue. Not all connective tissues are fascia, but all fascia is connective tissue. It can be thought of as a body-wide net that holds us together and is essential not just for our structure but also for the healthy functioning of our body. Paoletti describes fascia as "an uninterrupted, three-dimensional web of *tissue* that extends from head to toe, from front to back, from interior to exterior," showing us just how much it connects every part of our body.[6] The word *fascia* comes from the Latin and means "a band, bandage, swathe, ribbon,"[7] and in many ways this is a good description of the body's fascia, which does wrap our whole body, and is long, like a ribbon; so long it extends continuously from our head to our feet. You have probably already heard the word *fascia* used, possibly by a massage therapist or physiotherapist, in terms such as fascia lata or plantar fascia. Like the different seas, the different areas of fascia have their own names, but all are part of an interconnected whole. And not connected like the six-degrees-of-separation Kevin Bacon game. I mean completely connected. There are no free-floating pieces of fascia.

I believe that you also will have seen fascia before. You know that see-through filmy layer on chicken? That is fascia. Not all fascia is that fine and delicate, however; some is dense and strong, like the seam of tough white tissue that runs through steak. Hunters and butchers call it silverskin and it is very easy to see if you are skinning an animal.

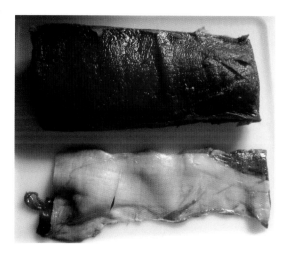

Figure 2.1 Hunters call fascia silverskin, which is easy to see on animals being skinned. Photograph courtesy of Public Land Hunters.

5 Lazier, 1943. 6 Paoletti, 2006. 7 Harper, 2016.

What the Fascia in Us Looks Like

There are several ways that we can look at fascia inside the body. None of them are very easy to do at home, but I have given examples here for your convenience.

1. CT

A CT (computed tomography) scan takes several X-ray images and makes them into one picture and is usually done to get a cross-sectional view of the body. In this cross-section of the abdomen, you can see that while organs and bones are very easy to spot, the fascia is not.

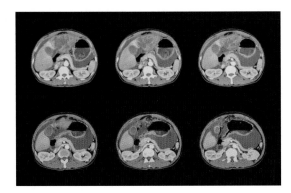

Figure 2.2 CT scan of the abdomen. Photograph courtesy of Shutterstock.

Even though the fascia is wide, wrapping the whole body and all of its structures, it is also shallow compared to other structures so it will always looks small or fine in cross-sectional images such as in CT scans or MRIs.

2. MRI

By using an MRI (magnetic resonance imaging) scan we can see a higher level of detail in the soft tissues including the fascia, in this case the plantar fascia (fascia on the sole of the foot). It creates an image by recording the effect of strong magnetic and radio waves on the millions of protons in our bodies, which react in different ways in the different tissues.

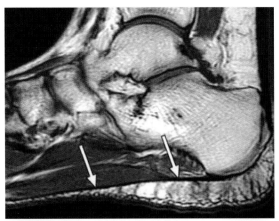

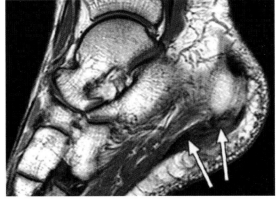

Figure 2.3 a) Healthy plantar fascia, and (b) severe plantar fasciitis. Photograph courtesy of Radsource.

As you can see the plantar fascia looks very smooth and streamlined in health, but after rupture it has thickened considerably (this is due to the growth of another type of tissue that is formed as a healing response to injury and is also built by fibroblasts, as the fascia is; in fact the fibroblasts have come from the nearby fascia in order to make it).

3. Ultrasound

Ultrasound bounces sound waves off things to see what they look like, similarly to the way dolphins and bats navigate. The sound is made by running electricity through quartz crystals, making them change shape quickly, vibrate, and produce a sound wave. The phenomenon of electricity affecting their structure is called piezoelectricity, discovered by Pierre and Jacques Curie in 1880[8] and although I do not think Pierre knew about the significance of fascia, I think he would have liked it, as fascia is also piezoelectric, courtesy of all the collagen in it—but I digress.

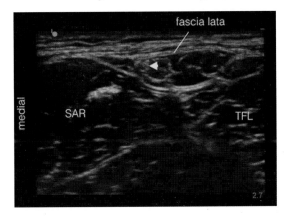

Figure 2.4 Ultrasound of fascia lata. Photograph courtesy of USRA.

In this ultrasound image of the front of the hip we can see the fascia lata, which wraps the thigh and hip muscles, as the denser, whiter area. You really need to know what you are looking for to spot the difference between muscle and fascia in ultrasound images.

4. Video Endoscopy

We can also pop a camera on a tube inside someone to look at their fascia up close (also known as video endoscopy). This is similar to putting a fiber optic camera underneath the doorways of criminals to see if they are armed before bursting in. We are not looking for guns, of course, but at the detailed structure of fascia in living people. This is quite different to that of the fascia of someone who is deceased, as you can observe it hydrated and moving rather than dry and inert.

Professor Jean-Claude Guimberteau uses this method to explore the unique geometric patterns within fascia. Looking at these two distinct images it is possible to see how fascia is organized differently in different areas of the body, depending on the function that is required of it. His videos are fascinating to watch (please see the resources section at the end of the book).

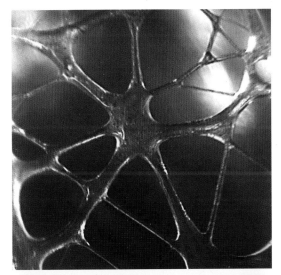

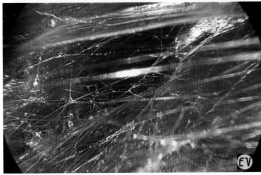

Figure 2.5 Video endoscopy of fascia.

8 Freudenrich, 2001.

5. Dissection

If Professor Guimberteau is the master of observing the fascia in the living, Gil Hedley is the wizard of observing the fascia after life, through dissection. His videos are enthralling and will give you a much better insight into the nature of fascia as a substance than a diagnostic scan will.[9]

The fact that dissections of fascia are being done at all is quite amusing since historically in a dissection the fascia would have been pushed aside and discarded having been considered irrelevant. It is now thought by many to be one of the most interesting parts of the body. If the early anatomists knew how fervently many people were now studying fascia they might well scratch their heads (hopefully without a scalpel in their hands). I was lucky enough to attend a dissection with Bowen teacher Julian Baker, to study the anatomy of the fascia within the body. Looking at the vast network of fascia and seeing just how interconnected the whole body's fascia is, confirmed to me the importance of working with it, whether through stretching or performing bodywork. This is because without affecting the fascia, there can be no improvement in structure or function.

It was also amazing to see just how different the state of the fascia is from one person to the next, shaped by their unique genes, lifestyle and movement patterns. Seeing the fascia within a body is one of the best ways of exploring the pervasive, sometimes strong and sometimes delicate network of fascia that exists throughout the body.

Dissection is also how Tom Myers came to discover the pathways within the fascia that connect the structures of the body functionally. They are known as Anatomy Trains, and this amazing system is the main theoretical model of the fascia used by bodyworkers today.[10]

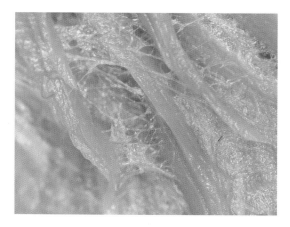

Figure 2.6 Dissection of fascia. Photograph courtesy of Julian Baker.

So if seeing is believing, I hope you now understand how interesting, important and "undeniably there" fascia is.

Why you May Not Have Heard of it Before

"What on earth is this and why have I not heard of it already?" seems to be the most common response from people I speak to about fascia. If it was that important, surely someone would have told you about it at work, at the gym or in the pub?

Well, the chances are that when you were at school your teachers did not know it was a big deal, or that the view of fascia would shift so much, from seeing it as an inert wrapping for your muscles and other structures, a sort of "plastic wrap for your body," to a completely integrated system that does so much more than holding bits in place. It does that as well, acting as a kind of scaffolding for the body, but imagine scaffolding that can give back-up strength, change shape as needed whilst maintaining its supportiveness, regulate water supply, support moving structures, hold things up in the right place in spite of bouncing and jiggling, and even function as a communication network.

We have moved from viewing fascia merely as inert scaffolding toward something that seems to be almost an intelligent structure. So, if it is so very important, why have you still not come across it before? Well it is not particularly exciting-looking (unless you are a fascia enthusiast) and surgeons are usually focused on getting through it to the "good stuff", that is, the things that you can actually point at that obviously do something. We like to be able to point at definite "things" with satisfyingly demarcated edges and a specific function that we can evaluate. When it comes to continuous, interconnected, and (to the untrained eye) apparently unremarkable structures, we are sometimes not sure how to investigate them, as our philosophy of science leans toward the study of detached objects; it is easier to measure, define, and compare them and to fit that information into existing knowledge bases. This has even happened with dissections of fascia, creating shapes with the scalpel that are then named as if they are individual structures. Yet each part is completely enmeshed within the whole.[11]

So what on earth is the fascia? Is it an organ, a structure, a communication network? If we tried to create a three-dimensional representation of its function with everyday objects we might end up with a rather bizarre sculpture of bubble wrap, cups of water, suspension bridge cables, telephone wires, quarantine tents and plastic wrap, whereas the older view may have represented it simply as clear wrapping.

As the fascia is thought to do more and more than we initially believed, it moves more and more into the limelight and new theories of its functioning may help to explain how our bodies operate as one integrated whole. Speaking personally, I feel reassured by the fact that we are more than just a collection of separate parts, we have a living, adaptable structure that takes its cue for its shape from how we live and move. And like anything that wants to survive, adapt, thrive, evolve, and expand, whether it is a society, a company, or a body, it needs a structure that is supportive enough to maintain a certain level of organization and efficiency and yet is not so restrictive that it prevents growth. This is fascia in a nutshell. A substance, a structure, and a system all in one tidy package, in which we are packaged.

11 Baker, 2016.

What the Condition of your Fascia Means to you

So if we all have fascia, so what? What difference does the state of our fascia make to us? My long-suffering model consented to being wrapped in plastic wrap to show you!

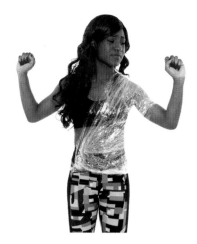

Figure 2.7A Tight fascia restricting movement.

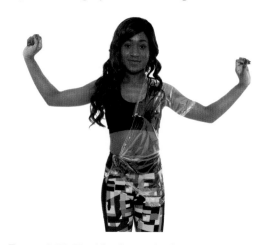

Figure 2.7B Healthy fascia facilitating normal movement.

Looking at these two photos, with the plastic wrap representing fascia, it is possible to see how built-up, thickened, and restrictive fascia can limit us, literally pulling us down. We have to actively use more force to move through that restriction, making everyday movements harder and more tiring than they should be. It is also very difficult to maintain good posture when your fascia is molded into a poor postural shape; as soon as you relax you are pulled straight back out of alignment.

12 Muscolino, 2012.

Some More Fascia Facts

I have been speaking about the fascia in quite general terms and this may already be enough information for you to start your stretching journey, but if you want to know more (or you have an analogy allergy) the facts and theories below may be useful to you.

We Have Three Main Types of Fascia

And they are:

1. superficial fascia

2. deep fascia

3. visceral (organ) fascia.

They are different by virtue of their location, function and composition.

The **superficial fascia** is, as its name suggests, closer to the surface of the body. It is also known as the hypodermis (hypo=under, dermis = skin).

It connects the skin to the deeper parts of the body and its structure is loose enough to allow for movement and flexibility in the skin. It is also more closely connected to the skin than to the deep fascia, to allow for more freedom of movement, so that the muscles can move separately to the skin. Its structure is like a honeycomb, but containing fat instead of honey.[12] This is important, because it ensures that we are able to stay warm and survive harsh winters or being submerged in cold water. Its flexibility also means that it can stretch to accommodate increased amounts of fat.

The **deep fascia** wraps around the muscles, bones, nerves, and blood vessels and it can create compartments that hold groups of muscles together.

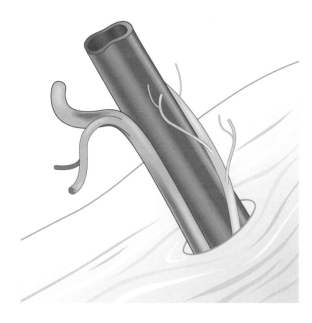

Figure 2.8 The superficial fascia will be perforated by structures such as arteries, veins, and nerves. (Illustration reproduced from Massage Fusion (Fairweather and Mari, 2015) with permission by Handspring Publishing)

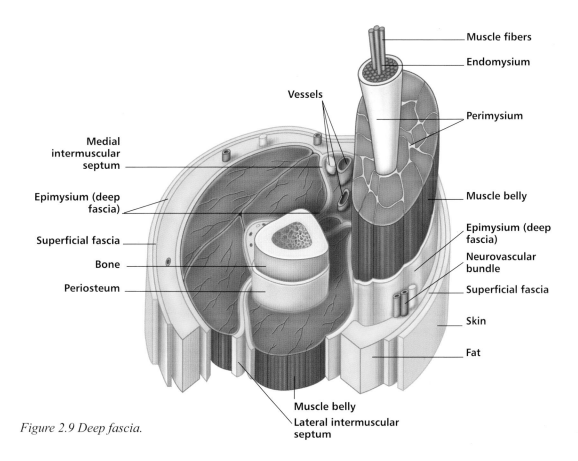

Figure 2.9 Deep fascia.

It is mainly the deep fascia that we affect when we stretch, and especially when we stretch with resistance. It is much tougher than superficial fascia and less flexible, but it is much more richly innervated (it is well supplied with nerves) and can report pain, movement, temperature, pressure, and chemicals in the environment around it.

Visceral fascia is responsible for holding the organs in their place, so it is the least stretchy type of fascia, but this is a good thing as if it stretches too much it leads to prolapse (organs dropping into places they should not be). The fibrous pericardium (the outer layer of the pericardium) is a great example of visceral fascia.

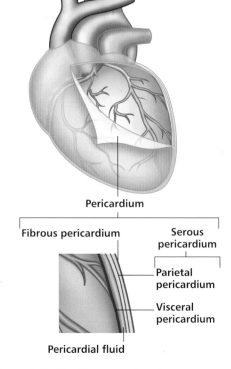

Figure 2.10 The fibrous pericardium, as an example of visceral fascia.

We want it to be flexible enough to allow our heart to beat, but tight enough to hold our heart in a protected and secure place so it does not bounce up and down when we run, for example. We do not focus on stretching the visceral fascia when we stretch, yet I believe that it can be affected positively through stretching.

What Fascia Is Made Of

Fascia is built out of three things:

1. collagen

2. elastin

3. ground substance

Let me use the metaphor of a well-functioning company to describe the jobs of these three building blocks of fascia. You have people who make the decisions and decide the structure (collagen), people who facilitate by being flexible and adapting as needed (elastin), and people who help by preventing friction between others and also other companies by facilitating communication, as well as providing what support is needed (ground substance). The proportions, structures, and qualities of these three materials in the fascia vary throughout the body, allowing the fascia to perform in the best way for each particular area. Whether it needs to be more rigid and structured, more flexible, more lubricated and slidey, or more sticky, the form that the fascia takes shapes our physical selves and that in turn is shaped by how we use our bodies.

Collagen is a protein, and the most abundant one in our body. It acts like scaffolding to provide strength and structure, which is an essential quality in the fascia. Without collagen we would look more like a puddle than a person, so our ability to move, interact with and affect our environment is very dependent on the collagen in our bodies.

Elastin, as its name suggests, is elastic in nature. It helps our tissue to stretch and move and be adaptable, which is most desirable in the superficial fascia and least desirable in the visceral fascia (do you want your heart bouncing up and down like a yoyo when you run?) and this is reflected in how much elastin they have. Deep fascia is somewhere in the middle, with varying amounts of elastin according to its location and what is required of it. Elastin does not just make our tissue elastic, like a rubber band, but also bendy, like our ears. Without elastin we would be more brittle and much easier to break.

Ground substance is a much more approachable name for "gluey interfibrillar proteins" or even "gylcosaminoglyans and proteoglycans," which it is made of as well as water. It is a see-through gelatinous substance said to look like raw egg-whites, with molecules in it that can absorb loads of water. It carries nutrients to cells, removes their waste products, and stops collagen fibers from rubbing against each other. It also helps the immune system by stopping bacteria from moving about freely.[13]

The fluid in most of our joints (synovial fluid) is one form of ground substance. It can be more slippery and lubricating when needed, or more sticky and holding, and also gets more fluid when it is warmer, and more solid when it is cooler, a property called "thixotropy".[14]

That is definitely enough grounding in fascia to get you started, but there is some more in depth information below, in case you are interested.

Fascia Has a Special Structure

Although it looks like a fairly inert, continuous flat sheet in most dissection photos, fascia actually has a very interesting shape and structure, which allows it to be strong, absorb force and lengthen or expand as needed. The shape of the fascia is different in different areas according to its function. In some places the fibers are arranged in a completely random, disorganized pattern and, in other places in an organized, or even fractal, pattern. A fractal is a repeating pattern which repeats self-same patterns at different scales (they also occur in lightning, peacocks, and trees, for example).

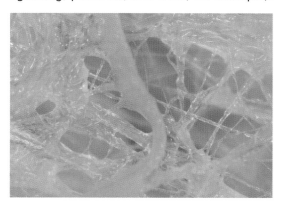

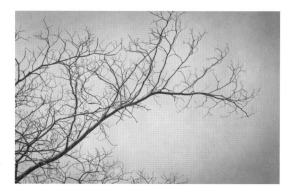

Figure 2.11 Fractal shape in (a) fascia (photograph courtesy of Julian Baker) and (b) a tree.

Along with the other tissues of the body, the fascia forms what is known as a tensegrity structure. The word tensegrity is made up of the words "tension" and "integrity" and was coined by Buckminster Fuller, an architect, and president of Mensa (he also created a number of other terms including "Spaceship Earth" and popularized the geodesic dome). The tensegrity structure pictured was constructed for the Burning Man gathering and represents the biomechanics of a human cell.

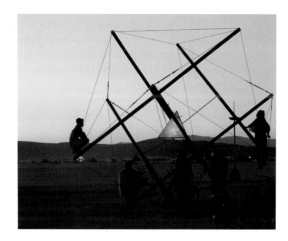

Figure 2.12 Tensegrity structure at Burning Man gathering. Photograph courtesy of Will Buchanan and the Tensegrity crew.

It is amazing that a part of our body as small as a cell may use tensegrity to maintain its shape and for other key functions.[15] The pattern of tensegrity being fundamental to our structure at both the minute and whole-

13 Myers, 2014. 14 Fritz, 2013. 15 Ingber, 2003.

body levels seems to mirror the fractal nature of fascia.

One of the first people to create tensegral structures, Kenneth Snelson, termed them "floating compression" structures, which reflects the fact that all the hard, rigid bits (also known as "spacers") are floating and do not touch each other and the continuous material that joins them up (also called the "tensional element"), is under a continuous tension, maintaining the integrity of the structure through that force.

Dr Stephen Levin coined the term *biotensegrity* to refer to this principle in anatomy.[16] In the body, the bones and cartilage are the spacers and the fascia is the tensional element.[17] This unique shape and structure gives the body its strength, resilience, and elasticity.

Fascia is Built By Fibroblasts

A fibroblast is a cell that makes collagen. If collagen molecules are the bricks of our fascial structure, then the fibroblasts are the builders. They are interesting because to do a particular job they have to change shape (almost as builders need different tools for different jobs) and they can also change shape as a response to acupuncture (for example, they become large and flat near inserted acupuncture needles), massage, and sustained stretching (up to 30 minutes).[18] It is amazing how alive and adaptable our fascia is.

Fascia Senses Things

Initally it was thought that there were no nerves in the fascia, and therefore it had no sensation, but actually research has shown that it is very richly enervated (i.e., it has a lot of nerves in it), especially with sensory nerves.

People used to think that the main job of the nerves in fascia was to relay pain signals, but actually they send all kinds of different information to the brain. Many of the nerves help with proprioception, which is the ability to have spatial awareness of parts of ourselves, or ourselves in relation to the outside world, know how fast parts of us, or our whole bodies, are moving and how much effort we are putting into movement. For example, we have nerves in our plantar fascia (the fascia on the sole of the foot) that send feedback to our brains that helps us to balance.

Other types of nerves in fascia have been shown to send information about sensation, position, and movement. Stimulation of these nerves can have an effect on blood pressure, heart rate, and respiration, showing how nerves in the fascia also help the body to regulate itself by providing local information.[19]

So if you had any doubt that fascia was not just an inert wrapping for the body, it is clear from its enervation that it is actually a sensory organ—and a highly atuned one at that. Interestingly I have noted that my students who stretch regularly (around three times a week or more) have improved proprioception and coordination.

Fascia Talks

Because the fascia is the only thing in the body that connects everything, it makes a lot of sense to think that it may also serve as a communication network for the whole body. The messages sent through this network come in a variety of forms; chemical, cellular, piezoelectric, and nervous (to do with the nerves rather than anxious!) messages can all move through the fascia. This may explain how a distant part of the body can affect another so strongly, or how we can react faster at times than a normal "nerve-based" response would allow. There is a theory also that fascia's ability to conduct electricity is the physiological reason that energetic treatments such as acupuncture or healing may work. That is pretty controversial, with, very broadly speaking, scientists tending not to like the idea very much and some alternative practitioners liking it quite a lot.[20]

16 Levin, 2013. 17 Oschman, 2015. 18 Langevin, 2013. 19 Schleip, 2003. 20 Oschman, 2009.

Fascia Can Contract

We have all been taught that our strength comes from our muscles, that and downing large quantities of spinach. However, our fascial system is also thought to contribute greatly to our strength. It can contract, not quite like a muscle does, but it can become tense, lending us emergency bursts of great strength and speed. Christopher McDougall, in his book *Natural Born Heroes*, mentions our ability to train our fascia to be strong, powerful, and elastic regardless of our size or gender. This means we could have superior strength and endurance without having larger muscles or being bigger than our opponents or competitors.[21]

The most obvious evidence we have that fascia can contract actually occurs in illness, in conditions such as Dupuytren's contracture, where the fascia in the palm of the hand thickens and shortens, pulling one or more fingers in toward the palm, often leading to severe restrictions in movement.

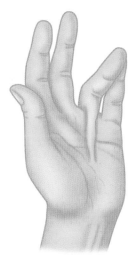

Figure 2.13 Dupuytren's contracture.

Frozen shoulder is another example of contraction in the fascia, one with no known cause. It is very interesting that in a frozen shoulder, the fascia can go from rigid and fixed back to moveable and elastic within a few days, spontaneously. However (more out of interest than to boast) I have stretched people with frozen shoulders that have not responded to other therapies and several people have experienced normal use and range of motion in their shoulder within 20–40 minutes. It just shows how quickly the fascia can respond, as long as we know how to work with it.[22]

Although it is easier to see fascia contracting in illness, it is believed to be able to contract in health because it contains contractile fibroblasts within it. This means that the fascia may play more than a passive role in the way the musculoskeletal system works. Again this is not a contraction like a muscle, but more of a stiffening effect, giving back-up strength through creating a stronger structure. It is amazing that something we once thought was an inert wrapping, is now thought to be able to actively influence musculoskeletal dynamics.[23]

Fascia Shapes Itself According to our Needs

Fascia seems almost intelligent as it can remodel itself in response to the demands we put on it. Through mechanotransduction (which means a mechanical force being converted into a signal) forces exerted on the tissue create a chemical response, often leading to physical changes. Force exerted on fascia can trigger collagen production and lead to changes in density, shape, or fiber arrangement in the fascia.[24]

On the healthy side, this is the mechanism of "use it or lose it." We create and improve our physical state through the way we move because the movement tells our body what we want it to become. However, it is worth noting that if we move too much and do not allow enough time for recovery, or our fascia is too tight, then we can produce too much collagen, leading to increased tension and restriction increasing our risk of injury.[25] Also if we repeatedly "tell" our fascia that we want to be the shape of people who hunch over for most of the day, it will also adapt to make us that way! So it is really important to keep moving and keep our movements natural and varied.

21 McDougall, 2015. 22 Schleip, Klingler & Lehmann-Horn, 2005. 23 Myers, 2014. 24 Kjaer, 2015. 25 Rodriguez, 2015.

We Need Just the Right Amount of Tension in our Fascia

As previously mentioned, movement leads to the production of collagen, creating sufficiently strong and dense fascia to support healthy movement and prevent instability and injury. One example of excessive flexibility causing injury is the higher likelihood of women to rupture their ACL (anterior cruciate ligament). Part of the cause may be hormonal, as at the time of the month when women are most flexible (when estrogen levels are highest) they produce 40% less collagen, which decreases the tensile strength of their ACL.[26]

However, excessive tension in the body and improper training can also lead to a build up of excess fascia. In order to be able to move fluidly and freely we need a fascial system that allows us the full use of our natural range of motion. This differs from person to person, but an obvious example of restriction due to excess fascia is the weightlifter who does not balance his lifting with mobility exercises. This can lead to restriction and pain and can only be remedied by restoring full range of motion.[27]

The amount of fascia that each person has is individual to their bodies and their lifestyles and we discuss this in more depth in Chapter 5 (Why Some People Aren't Stretchy (and Others Are).

Fascia Distributes Force Throughout the Body

Because the fascia forms an interconnected network encompassing all of the body's structures, when a force affects one part of the body, the fascia automatically acts as a kind of shock-spreader-and-absorber. It also distributes this force within the body, as when we contract our muscles the force is distributed through the muscle and fascial network, which is thought to be the way that muscular force moves from one muscle to another. One of the foremost experts in research on fascia, Dr Robert Schleip, who discovered the active contractile properties of fascial tissues, has described the fascia as being part of "a body-wide tensional force transmission system."[28]

Fascia Stays More Youthful if Hydrated

I bet you did not know that there was a difference between fascia that is more youthful and fascia that is aging. The difference is that the younger-feeling fascia is more elastic, springy, strong (in older children and adults rather than babies, in whom it is softer) and hydrated, whereas if it is aging it can become less elastic, tighter, frayed and dried out. So how do you get water into the fascia? The answer is through movement and physical interventions such as stretching, massage and foam rolling, and then to rest. This is because when you are using the body, you are squeezing the tissues like a sponge being wrung out and when you rest, the fascia can suck up more water and become hydrated.[29]

I hope some of these facts help you to understand why it is so important that we take care of our fascia and give it a regular stretching spring-clean.

Now that we have had a pretty thorough look at fascia, let us look at how it feels about being stretched.

26 Silvers and Mandelbaum, 2007. 27 Starrett, 2015. 28 Schleip et al., 2012. 29 Myers, 2012.

Resistance Stretching and the Fascia

Resistance stretching really is the new kid on the block of the stretching scene in terms of being an official technique; most people have never heard of it and it does not even have its own Wikipedia entry yet. Usually when I mention it people think it may have something to do with resistance bands (the stretchy bands used for strength training). (It doesn't by the way, although we do occasionally use yoga straps.) By way of a brief explanation I often describe it as "a system of stretching that works on the fascia by tensing the muscles and then moving the body against that resistance." But we can do better than that. Let us start by looking at how animals do it.

Stretching for Pandas

As previously mentioned, animals have a very powerful and instinctive way of stretching. When a big cat decides that she has had enough of lying around she will get up slowly and go right into a resistance stretch. This means that she does not just relax back into child's pose, sitting back on her haunches serenely with her head touched to the floor. Instead, she pulls her front paws forcefully down into the ground, tensing her whole body as she sticks her bottom out behind and pushes her chest down to the floor. This movement against tension is a form of resistance stretching and in natural movement circles is also known as *pandiculation*.

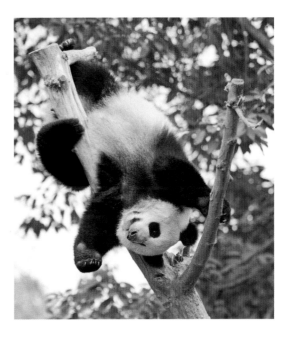

Figure 3.1 Panda stretching (pandiculation)!

Pandiculation is not actually a panda-specific exercise (although pandas do like to do it!). The word comes from the Latin *pandiculari*, which means "to stretch oneself" and mainly refers to the short, more intense, and instinctive stretches in animals and also in humans when yawning. It is a full-body stretch where you tense your muscles and move through that force, engaging the fascia and muscles and deeply awakening and stretching them, and therefore is a type of resistance stretching.

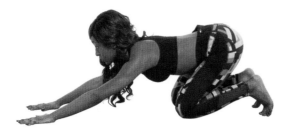

Figure 3.2 Stretching like a cat.

However, due to our socialization we do not do this very much, and especially not in public. We do like to have a context and a goal for what we are doing, which is why it is more comfortable for many of us to have a specific time set aside for stretching, unlike animals who often stretch every time they get up and all throughout the day.

Resistance Stretching for Humans

This is where pandiculation and resistance stretching differ; while the former is spontaneous, deep, and short, the latter can be done for longer periods of time, works more deeply into the body, and brings about specific long-term changes. The function of pandiculation is to warm the body up, to get the blood circulating, to prepare the muscles for movement, and to blow away the cobwebs that have built up after a period of inactivity. Resistance stretching does that too, but based on the results I have seen, I believe that it also goes beyond that, creating a deeper and more lasting change.

With Resistance Stretching We Can Work into our "Deep Tension"

By stretching for a longer time we can work through our "superficial tension" (that which has been created most recently and is easier to shift, and can be relieved by a quick minute of pandiculation, for example) into our "deep tension" (which has built up over months, years, or decades and is both deeper in the body as well as more intractable). Animals do not need to stretch much as they usually do not have the same type of deep tension that limits their movement; they do what they need to do physically, and which is natural to them, all day, every day.

The tension in their body, whether superficial or deep, is reflective of how they were built to move and actually helps them to make these movements easily, efficiently, and powerfully. Therefore, the shape of their fascia supports and boosts all of their daily movements. The only time that an animal would have tension limiting their movement would be if they had experienced a strong trauma to the body or had been living in cramped conditions, unable to move as their instincts guide them to.

We humans are much more than a hop, skip, and a jump away from our instincts, and more often than not an escalator ride, 8–14 hours of immobile sitting and 5 hours of smartphone or tablet use closer to a bizarre form of living rigor mortis, so we need a little more help. I blame the mind for a lot of it. Whereas animals let instinct guide them, aware and present in their bodies, we defer on most matters to the intellect and lose most (or all) awareness of anything beneath our eyeballs. We concentrate and hunch, tensing our shoulders and necks, and stay very still whilst fixated on one thing. Our fascia adapts to support us in this position, and then when we try to stand up tall or move freely, we have to actively pull against that built-up fascia. Working to release that restrictive fascia is the essence of resistance stretching.

Try this at home

Fancy a go? Let's do two very similar exercises, the first without resistance and the second with resistance. I want you just to keep an open mind and notice how you feel during and after each.

1. Without resistance (i.e., relaxed muscles), move your arms up above your head and out and down either side, in a wide arc.

2. Do the same but tense (or "squeeze") the muscles in your abdomen, chest, arms, and shoulders first and keep that tension going while you make the movement.

Which one was more relieving and had the strongest effect?

(If you are somewhere where you cannot wave your arms around, try doing a more subtle experiment. Move your shoulders as far forward and then as far back as you can, with your muscles relaxed/ normal, and then repeat with tension in your back and chest. I recommend that you give the full exercise a go when you can).

In terms of achieving our physical potential, the absolute ideal is to move throughout the day in a large variety of ways, most of which are currently socially unacceptable in the street or in the office, and to stretch spontaneously when the urge arises, in order to get the variety of movement our bodies need for healthy and strong tissue. This would train our fascia to keep us open, tall, functional, and healthy. However, this is difficult for many of us—we can crawl, squat, and jump at home, but may prefer not to in public. Because natural movement is confined to restricted times in the day for most people, we need a little extra help.

Stretching regularly with resistance to recondition our fascia can help to restore us to our natural freedom of movement. Clients and students have reported feeling lighter, freer, more youthful, taller, looser, and more graceful, and I have noticed that they seem to look younger, move better, and have better posture. Or, if you are one of the few who have the good luck to be able to move naturally for several hours a day, then resistance stretching will help you to improve on the solid foundation you are already building.

Resistance Stretching Increases Your Strength

Because resistance stretching is performed by lengthening a muscle, or group of muscles, whilst they are contracting (you could also say they are "tensed" or "resisting"), you are actually performing an "eccentric contraction," also known as a "lengthening

contraction" in yoga. When doing repetitions it is known as "eccentric training;" weight lifters also call it "negative training." In the context of general exercise it is used to strengthen the muscles as well as being a method of rehabilitating injured tendons. Weightlifters train this way for rapid gains in strength and muscle size as you can use heavier weights than you can lift normally and there is less neural inhibition (i.e., your nervous system does not get in the way as much).[30]

Muscles that are trained eccentrically also stay stronger for longer, as well as increasing in size (please bear in mind that weightlifters are using very heavy weights indeed, so you are not going to suddenly develop enormous muscles from resistance stretching). So if you do not have time to do your strength training and your flexibility training this may be a win–win for you. You can kill two birds with one stretch, proving that resistance is not futile! (no, I can't believe I wrote that either).

The "Resistance" in Resistance Stretching Helps to Increase Flexibility

Eccentric training has also been proven to boost flexibility through the creation of more sarcomeres (the stretchy bits in muscles, inside the myofibrils, mentioned earlier), simultaneously making a muscle both longer and stronger.[31] The main reason that we use resistance in resistance stretching, however, is to get the fascia involved. While it takes more of a back-seat role in many physical movements and functions, it really comes into its own in resistance stretching and eccentric strength training. The fact that fascia is now known to be an important player in musculoskeletal dynamics, supports the theory that it is "engaged" in eccentric strength movements, providing additional strength to support the muscles. We are trying actively to make it resist and we then use movement to work through any adhesions, limitations and even scar tissue in the area being stretched and beyond. Resolving these issues and re-conditioning the fascia has a great impact on flexibility, as long as there are healthy gains in range of motion to be made.

Resistance Stretching may be Safer than Static Stretching

Because of the eccentric nature of resistance stretching, Tom Myers believes that it is potentially safer than other forms of stretching due to the simultaneous in-series engagement of the muscles, fascia, ligaments, and tendons. By distributing the force evenly through all of the tissues during a stretch, we avoid accidentally over-straining specific areas. In other forms of stretching people relax their muscles so that they can go further in a stretch, but this puts a lot of the strain into the place where the tendon meets the bone (periosteum), often causing tendon-insertion injuries which can take ages to heal.[32]

Stretching while Moving May Help our Nervous System to Accept a Greater Range of Motion

Another thing that differentiates resistance stretching from other more passive forms of stretching is its effect on the nervous system. One aspect of this is that when we are moving actively our nervous system learns how to support our limbs and torso in certain positions, that is, in greater ranges of motion, much more so than when we move more passively. Therefore active movement is likely to boost performance more than more passive stretching modalities.[33] This is another aspect of "use it or lose it," as in "use your entire range of motion or soon you won't be able to," and it explains why incorporating movement into every single stretch is part of what makes resistance stretching so effective (and Moving Stretch® in particular, which incorporates movement into each and every stretch).

You are More Stable when you Resistance Stretch

In my experience in the clinic and classroom I have seen that, because resistance stretching strengthens you at the same time as stretching you, you maintain much more stability in your body. This is especially important around your joints, because it is the correct balance of tension and freedom of movement that allows your joints to function efficiently and safely.

Stability and integrity are so important that gains in flexibility without maintaining stability are not really gains at all but a liability. Engaging your muscles and strengthening them at the same time as you engage your fascia and stretch ensures that you are not just pulling at your body to make it longer, but making sustainable increases in flexibility that are balanced by strength.

Eccentric, or "lengthening" contractions occur as a natural aspect of yoga practice, whenever a person lowers themselves or a limb with control and also during more challenging poses.[34] The benefits include moving with control, protecting the body in poses that might otherwise lead to strain and also longer-lasting increases in range of motion.

It is Like Bodywork that you Do to Yourself

Because we move through the whole range with resistance, we are also combing through the tissue, working on it a little like a body worker does, but from the inside. How cool is that? We can shift any stuck bits (adhesions), work into tight areas, help to re-hydrate the tissue, boost blood circulation, and flush out the toxins being held in the tissue, all just by moving with a bit of resistance. I believe that you can clean yourself out from the inside.

You Start Looking Younger

Say what? Yes, all of the clients I have ever worked with who stretch regularly two to three times a week look younger than they did when they started, even if they started years ago. It really seems to counter and prevent unnecessary aging (actually, much of what many consider to be the normal signs of aging I think of as being unnecessary; see Chapter 5 for more information). This is due to the reconditioning of your fascia allowing your state and shape to be closer to your original blueprint than the roadmap

32 Myers, 2016. 33 Lederman, 2015. 34 Coulter, 2010.

of stress, late nights, and inactivity we create through being a human in the 21st century. Let us take all that tense and tired fascia out, and look like ourselves again!

It Plays Well With Others

Resistance stretching is an amazing addition to your exercise routine. It helps performance, improves the quality of your movements, increases strength and flexibility, boosts energy and posture, and is a great way of approaching a "problem' from another angle (for example, a specific movement or pose that was not improving through repeatedly doing it). Moving Stretch® has helped people improve in their yoga, running, climbing, cycling, dancing, and even on expeditions and more. It does not need to replace your usual physical activities, it can boost them instead, hopefully making them easier, more satisfying and enjoyable.

All of the Things That Make Resistance Stretching a Little Bit Different (or a LOT)

I want to quickly reiterate the major differences between resistance stretching and other types of stretching and movement techniques, as I know it can be hard to get our heads around a new technique sometimes.

The Resistance Part

As far as I know, no other stretching or techniques use resistance like this, they only use it at or near the end of the range of motion. For example, you would go to the end of the range and then create tension, but not move through the whole range against tension. Therefore it is unlikely that other stretching techniques have the same effect on fascia that resistance stretching has, though they will of course affect it to some degree.

It Involves Movement

Most of the stretches involve moving through a whole range of motion, rather than going right to the end and pushing to increase that. With resistance stretching the stretch only occurs within the existing healthy range of motion, and even though we stay within this, the ROM can still increase if it is helpful for the body. This reflects the fact that the cause of inflexibility may just not be that one muscle or group of muscles cannot lengthen enough, but that there may be adhesions, tension, or dehydration in the fascia, weakness in the muscles and, or resistance in the nervous system, which is limiting your range of motion. Stretching with movement can help to address these issues.

We Get Fast Results

Working on the fascia in addition to the muscles, instead of only focusing on the muscles, produces excellent results. Don't get me wrong, focusing on the muscles is great and, of course, it is impossible to affect the muscles without also affecting the fascia. However, by working in a way that engages and reconditions the fascia specifically, you are affecting the framework of the body directly, rather than just working on separate little pieces. That is a powerful tool.

The Results Can Be Very Long Term

At a very rough guess I would say that my clients keep around 70% of the benefits of their stretching afterwards, but this varies according to the individual (their lifestyle, tissue quality, health, diet, etc.) and the issue being worked on. For beginners I expect that if they do the stretching three times a week for 2 months they may get some changes that will last for 6–12 months and other changes that will wear off without further stretching. I know that is a very broad estimate, but there are huge differences according to the person's tissue and lifestyle. For example if you sit hunched at a desk 5 days a week, then you will need to continue to stretch to "unhunch" yourself for as long as that is the case.

A Body for All Seasons

I have noticed that my students who stretch regularly have healthier, more resilient and adaptable bodies, even though most of them do different sports and have different lifestyles. This suggests to me that resistance stretching is a good form of conditioning that can support other activities and a healthy lifestyle.

That Fascia Stuff

Fascia works hard for the body, protects us, and does its best to keep us working as a well-functioning whole, often in spite of our best efforts to hurt ourselves with poor posture, binge exercising, or sitting marathons. However, it is only recently that its importance has been noted. Where many therapies are now only just incorporating this information, working on the fascia has been one of the core principals of resistance stretching since it began. It takes a very specific approach to affect fascia in a positive way. Because it is in charge of maintaining our form (shape) it does not like to be randomly pulled about, because there is nothing random about the structure and function of our body. It has all been shaped by design and conditioning, and ways of working with our body should be by design too.

So, to sum up, the mechanism of resistance stretching is different to other stretching, exercise, and movement techniques because of its greater involvement of the fascia (which stretches differently to muscles), the simultaneous contraction and lengthening of the muscles, its active nature, and its shorter (safer) range of motion. Because of this, resistance stretching offers unique benefits, beyond that which you might expect from stretching.

What Moving Stretch Is

All of the schools of resistance stretching, aside from differences in technique or theory, use tension in the muscles to engage the fascia and tend to move through almost the whole range of motion from beginning to end, whether moving a limb or the whole body. Moving Stretch® is no exception.

After originally training in resistance stretching with Bob Cooley in Boston, MA, I went on to practice for several years and then to develop my own method, based on what I had found to be the most effective and accessible for my clients, who were often novices to stretching as well as time poor. My clients had unique individual flexibility and strength needs, depending on their bodies and lifestyles. I realized that a simple and flexible, yet effective, system could be adapted to suit the needs of each individual, even though the desired end result was different. For example, a dancer and a builder can both use Moving Stretch® to increase their strength and flexibility to support the ways they need to be able to move and function because it is "self-tailoring" to each individual body. The range of motion is the distance that you can go comfortably, the level of resistance is dictated by the strength in your own muscles, and how much you do depends on your energy levels and how your body feels at the time. No two bodies are the same and this system was designed accordingly.

I named the method Moving Stretch® because it is the movement aspect of the technique that is the magic ingredient, boosting people's health, vitality, and freedom to move. A very simple technique, it does not require hours of study to get started, only a brief introduction, in a class or through this book, and somewhere convenient to stretch. It is made up of individual stretches (Moving Stretches) that work on different areas of the body as well as stretching routines that benefit our fascia and our bodies as a whole, boosting flexibility, strength and health.

The popularity of resistance stretching is growing along with the interest in fascia, and whereas in the past it may have been reserved for the elite athlete or very wealthy individual, Moving Stretch® is for people from all backgrounds who want to experience a stronger and freer body and enjoy themselves while they do so. I hope you do too!

A New Look at Stretching and Flexibility

Does Stretching Always Mean Going Further and Does Flexibility Mean Doing the Splits?

What is stretching, really? Is it a movement? Is it going right to the end of our range of motion and trying to push beyond it? Is it staying in a specific pose? And what is flexibility: the ability to do the splits, bend over backward, or touch our toes? Can we say that a ballet dancer is flexible and a builder is not?

These are questions we would rarely ask, because the answers may seem so obvious. Yet with the rise in interest and controversy around stretching (especially in bodywork and exercise circles), it is important that we look at what we will be doing and what we can achieve through resistance stretching.

Static stretching, where we go to the end of our range of motion (ROM) and try to push further beyond it, is the method we were taught in school and the first thing that most people think of when considering increasing their flexibility. Unfortunately, static stretching has been shown to actually impair performance, especially in those sports requiring more elastic recoil and efficiency of movement, such as sprinting,[35] and can even increase the risk of injury.

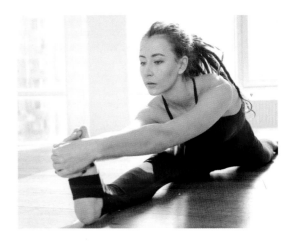

Figure 4.1 Stretching should not be a no-pain, no-gain activity.

Forcing our muscles and fascia to lengthen by pushing beyond pain and our natural range of motion does not lead to healthy lasting change. Stretching, at its best, is a natural and healthy way of moving that increases our ability to move with power and grace within ranges of motion that are useful to us. Pushing ourselves out of this range I would therefore call over-stretching, as it goes beyond that which is useful and may lead to strain and injury. If you want to increase your range of motion for a specific goal, such as doing the splits, for example, you must also make sure that you are strong throughout the entire range, so that it is safe for your body.

35 Marek et al., 2005.

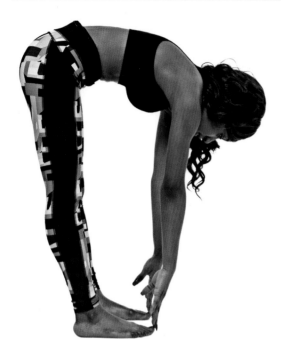

Figure 4.2A In static stretching you try to increase flexibility by reaching further.

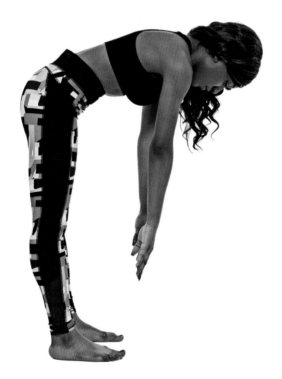

Figure 4.2B In resistance stretching you stretch within your natural range of motion.

Resistance stretching is very different to static stretching in that we do not try to push into a range of motion where we do not have enough strength to support ourselves. It can

actually strengthen us at the same time as we stretch, and because it boosts strength alongside flexibility, I believe it would not have the same detrimental impact on performance that static stretching does.

The older paradigm of thinking that a larger range of motion is always better is outdated and can be harmful to us. There is often a price to pay, whether that price is that a part of our bodies becomes too loose to function properly, becomes unstable or loses elasticity, that our power, strength, or balance is impaired, or even that we develop a strain or more serious injury; sometimes our bodies do not want or need to go further in the way we think they should.

You may respond with examples of gymnasts, dancers, and practitioners of other movement-based disciplines, who have (and need for their sport) a larger range of motion. All of those people not only stretched to achieve and maintain that range, they used it, and by doing so, strengthened their bodies throughout that whole movement. This ensures that the greater range of motion is not only useful, but safe, because no single part has to bear the brunt of the effort; the muscles, ligaments, tendons, and fascia have all been conditioned and can all keep up with the demands made upon them. Because they continue to use that range of motion, they are much more likely to maintain it without straining themselves.

However, when other people see that this level of flexibility is possible they often try to achieve it for themselves through (over-) stretching; pushing beyond their natural range without strengthening through that range also. This often leads to "pulling" on the weaker areas rather than the tight areas that need it most, instability in the joints, imbalance in the body, and an increased likelihood of strain and injury. In addition the body will not prioritize keeping a range of motion that is not used regularly and will let it shrink again, in which case the only remedy is to keep up regular stretching exercises to maintain it. The only plus side of stretching in this way is that if someone is very sedentary or cannot do other exercise for various reasons, it does give them access to some form of movement, which, generally speaking, is better than no movement at all. On the downside this is not the most useful approach for keeping ourselves flexible as flexibility without strength and structure is not flexibility at all, but a liability.

Thinking about stretching only as a way to increase our range of motion, without any thought to strength, the quality of our tissue, what movements are useful to us, our body structure, and other factors, is similar to overhauling your car in every way possible to make it able to go faster, whilst neglecting to upgrade the engine. It is a flawed strategy.

Where Does Stretching End and Movement Begin?

A different point of view, which I have only heard expressed in circles of movement and alternative health specialists and never by the general public, is that stretching is at best useless and at worse downright harmful. I believe this does come down to what we consider stretching, vs over-stretching, to be. Above, I described the importance of having a useful range of motion that we are strong in and can use, rather than an increased range just for the sake of it, and most arguments against stretching come down to this one point.

Where stretching ends and movement begins, is a little blurred, however, and as all of the stretches in this book involve movement and healthy ranges of motion, I believe it is in line with the philosophy of many other movement and remedial techniques and in practice works very well in conjunction with them.

Many would argue that if we can obtain the same result simply by moving more, why wouldn't we? Well, if we lived in a world where we could feasibly move naturally in healthy and organic ranges of motion for around 6 hours a day, unfettered by office work, electronic devices, and social norms I would probably have to restrict my work to those who had been involved in accidents or other unusual circumstances and needed special help, because everyone else would be healthy and open and tall. This would

be wonderful and I would be for it, even if I would be out of a job! But, because many of us have to use a computer for hours, sit down, behave ourselves in public and are restricted in a million other ways, it makes sense to use a method that is like movement $\times$ 2. Because, although resistance stretching is not a replacement for healthy, natural movement, you can use it to help you catch up to where you would be if you had not been sitting all day.

This is due to the fact that the resistance makes it much more powerful and at a very rough guess I would say that doing 25 minutes of resistance stretching leads to the same improvement in posture and quality of movement as an hour or more of more gentle movement. If you have time for movement as well as resistance stretching you will get even better results, and many of my clients who are dancers, athletes, and other types of movers have found that it maximizes their performance and enjoyment of their other physical activities.

However, if people can only fit in 10–20 minutes for movement a day, then resistance stretching can do a lot to help undo the damage created by lack of movement. Simply put, it helps to release us from the torpor and physical stagnation of a day at the office.

How Much Can You Change Through Stretching?

As I have said before, this is a strong form of stretching, working on the body's fascia as well as increasing physical strength. In a way it is like bodywork that you do to yourself. You may use it to temporarily relieve tightness or pain, or as part of your workout routine, but I want you to know that if you commit to a regular stretching practice you can expect amazing results. Try not to limit your stretching to a very specific need or time only (such as in the gym), but take the time to fully explore the benefits it can offer you by putting in a bit more time on a regular basis and trying a variety of stretches.

I have already spoken about the benefits of stretching and the changes I have seen in my clients. The most remarkable ones have been almost like watching a person come back to life as the shine returns to their eyes, their thinking becoming clearer and their movements more definite, smooth, and refined; almost as if their consciousness was increasing in focus and brightness and their body was returning to its natural state of strength, grace, and openness.

I may be waxing lyrical because I am a stretching trainer, but I have seen amazing transformations take place. My clients often experience improvements in their posture, the way they hold themselves, even added height. This photo was taken after four 1-hour assisted stretching sessions over 4 weeks (I stretched the client rather than him stretching himself, but these changes can also occur through self-stretching, especially if people are stretching daily rather than just once a week).

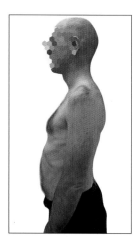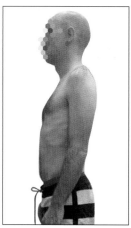

Figure 4.3 Client-before and after.

As you can see, his posture has improved considerably; his ribs stick out much less, his upper back is much less hunched, and his hips are less flexed (you can tell because his stomach is flatter). I believe that the change in these photos illustrates just how crucial it is to recondition the fascia and stretch and strengthen the muscles if you want to improve posture.

Interestingly, some clients also become better looking, with more distinct and clear features. I myself transformed physically through stretching and when I show people photographs of myself, they cannot believe how much I have changed.

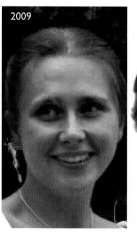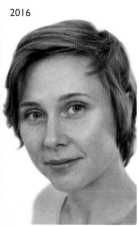

Figure 4.4 Then and now.

It is not just a loss of body fat, but a "remodeling" of my fascia, which took the heaviness and padding out of my face (also called "armouring") which you can see from the noticeable change in shape. My friends and colleagues of the same age have not changed anywhere near that much in 7 years (nor do they need to!). It is different to the before and after photos a nutritionist or personal trainer would take. I believe that some people have more potential to change in this way through stretching than others because they start off with a greater amount of tight, restrictive or built-up fascia. As we focus on the fascia as the medium that can change, we can remove this excess, restoring the body to its potential. This is my theory based on what I have observed in my teaching and private practice. It will be interesting to see what information research can add to this area in the future, beyond resistance stretching's ability to "clean up" the arrangement of fibers within the fascia.

Ways of Working on the Fascia

There are several other techniques that lead to amazing benefits, such as myofascial release, structural integration (also known as Rolfing), and Bowen technique, for example, which specifically work on the fascia. But in addition to these, any other physical technique that benefits the body will affect the fascia by default, whether or not it targets it specifically.

My clients who are yoga teachers and students have a very nice quality tissue, which feels oxygenated, spongy, and elastic. Because teaching yoga is a very physical job, the teachers very occasionally come to me with strains, especially near joints, but for the most part their fascia has adapted well to the demands placed upon it and has strength, flexibility, and integrity. The only minor point I would make is that the bodies of yoga practitioners can sometimes be a little weaker when going off specific lines of motion, which I believe is due to sticking to a very specific alignment in the poses. I think the addition of some more general and varied movements, maybe once a week for example, could improve the structural integrity and functioning of the fascia in all ways, as well as its strength.

Some of the nicest and healthiest tissue I have worked with is in people who (by design or by chance) have a rich variety of movement in their lives, especially those using natural movement techniques. This usually involves the basics of human movement, including squatting, jumping, climbing, lifting and throwing, and doing it as efficiently and gracefully as possible.

Another natural form of movement that is experiencing a resurgence in popularity is the barefoot running movement. Galahad Clark, who runs the barefoot shoe company Vivobarefoot, believes that running barefoot (or in minimal shoes) allows us to move naturally, while lots of cushioning and structure in shoes "deprives the brain of the information it needs to control natural, healthy movement patterns."[36] Because people are not relying on the shoes to provide the "bounce," this must come from within their bodies, so in effect they train their fascia to provide the elastic force they need to run. From my experience, this produces nice quality, strong, and elastic fascia. Most people need to build up to running longer distances in barefoot-style shoes, however, as most of us have worn structured shoes from a young age.

In his book *Natural Born Heroes*, Christopher McDougall explains that the superior endurance, strength and movement technique of the people of Crete is due to their conditioning of, and harnessing the power of, the fascia. His theory was that they had trained it over their lifetime by quickly traversing their homeland's mountainous and sometimes treacherous terrain, an endeavor requiring "springiness," strength, and endurance in the body, which their fascia had adapted to provide them with. This is an example of how the fascia can be trained and conditioned to reinforce the structure and function of the body.

I myself had an early experience of working with my fascia that could be seen as pretty much the opposite of the mountain goat-like people of Crete. I started to do Tai Chi every week for 2 hours when I was 16 years old, and continued this for 2 years. Through slow and graceful movements I was building up patterns of movement within my fascia that I believe have remained to this day. About 15 years later I was walking from a train with a cup of tea in one hand and texting with my phone in the other (yes, I know, but I'm self-employed and it's the only way I can stay on top of my admin!). A taller, larger man running for the train I had just got off, ran at me full tilt, and without my even looking up my body reacted reflexively by moving my arm quickly out in a circular motion. The full-grown man was flung to the side and he bounced off a wall before shaking his head, slightly dazed, and then running for the train again. By the time this had all occurred I was just beginning to look up and notice what had happened. My body had not felt the force of it at all; I was exactly where I had been and my whole body felt relaxed, as if I had not tensed one muscle. So there are definite benefits to conditioning your fascia!

Of course, fascia was not a "thing" back when I started working with it. All I had was my friendly Tai Chi teacher, Raj, reminding me to stay relaxed, and later a rotund and powerful Tai Chi master swatting at me with (I hope mock) anger, telling me over and over not to use my muscles. A conundrum, keep my arms up without using muscle, so use

36 Hurley, 2012.

what then? Fascia. Through maintaining a stance or moving, whilst keeping our muscles out of it, we conditioned our fascia through repetitive gentle movements to make fast, reflexive movements that are helpful in self-defense (and at train stations!). We harnessed the power of fascia: to maintain a posture for a long time, to give our chosen structure a great amount of strength to withstand external force, and to inject rocket fuel into our pushes and punches.

What about Bruce Lee's 1-inch punch? Yes, he harnessed the power of fascia. Kung Fu, a kissing cousin of Tai Chi, recruits the power of fascia to the maximum, practitioners even using it to prevent spears from piercing their throats in one of their displays of superior "self-dominance" (to paraphrase Ido Portal, a natural movement expert who seems to have conditioned his fascia excellently).

I can feel the difference in the quality of people's fascia when I stretch them with resistance, in assisted stretching sessions. In those with conditioned and strong fascia, their bodies are receptive, adapt quickly, and understand what to do with the force I am putting in to change their fascia. When I stretch more sedentary people, their fascia feels compartmentalized and their strength fragmented, they find it harder to engage it by creating resistance and it is hard for them to use the force I am putting in. I believe that this is because people who have already learned how to harness the power of their fascia naturally understand how to use the force of resistance to engage it.

What has all this got to do with stretching the fascia? I want you to really understand the implications of working with your fascia, so that when you stretch you know that you are working with the architecture of your body and that can be a powerful thing. The quality of people's tissue even seems to improve with resistance stretching, becoming higher quality, more spongy, oxygenated, resilient, and youthful. I notice this in my one-on-one clients whose tissue I feel through walking massage and stretching them. I put this down to the fact that the whole body is engaged and affected by a resistance stretching session.

Because of this, it is sensible to only stretch with good technique, respect for your body and awareness of what is going on. So often in the West we approach our bodies as a manager would approach an under-performing department. Except that the only thing that can underperform is us, in our decision of how to treat our body. Our bodies are constantly working for us, even though often underappreciated, and we should treat them with this in mind. When they are tight, or break down, it is not their fault ("stupid shoulder!") but ours ("maybe I should take better care of myself, move more naturally and train sensibly"). It may seem like a minor point, but the way we think of our bodies has a huge effect on the way we train, stretch and treat ourselves.

Where healthy and useful, your range of motion will increase through resistance stretching. The positive thing about resistance stretching, is that it requires quite a lot of strength for each stretch, therefore in some ways it is harder to over-stretch yourself as you will usually fatigue before then. This even goes for naturally strong people. However, it is still possible to overdo it, especially by stretching intensely before warming up, so please read How to Stretch (Chapter 9) before you begin.

I hope this chapter has given you some food for thought, and maybe even slightly altered the way you see flexibility and stretching and their purpose. As humans, part of our birthright is to live, move, breathe, and be free. Too much strength without flexibility and we transform into little henchmen without necks, that cannot move. Too much flexibility without strength and we flop down at the first gust of wind and cannot open jars.

True physical freedom, therefore, is having both the full range of motion and the power to move through it with strength and grace. Useful stretching promotes this balance within you, leading to genuine, sustainable flexibility.

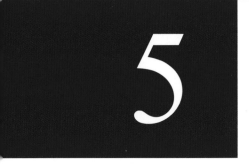

5

Why Some People Aren't Stretchy (and Others Are)

It seems so unfair that some people can easily tuck a leg behind their head while others struggle to touch their toes, or even get their fingers down past their knees. You probably already know whether you are a flexible person or not. You may have been naturally supple as a child, have pursued and enjoyed activities such as gymnastics or dance, and may still have good, or above average, flexibility. At the other end of the scale, you may remember not being able to touch your toes as a teenager, feeling tight and inflexible for a lot of your life, and now describe yourself as "stiff as a board," or as one person put it, "about as flexible as a house brick." The majority are on a spectrum somewhere between these two extremes.

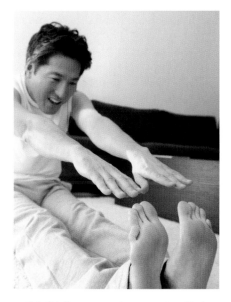

Figure 5.1 (b) Some people are naturally less flexible. Photograph courtesy of Shutterstock.

So why are some people more stretchy than others? We are going to take a look at genetics, age, gender, health, diet, and other lifestyle factors. Hopefully this will give you a clue as to how you can optimize your life for flexibility.

Is it in Your Genes?

First, let us take a look at a group one might consider naturally flexible, ballet dancers. A study found that two specific genotypes (your unique combination of genes) were more flexible than another genotype, within a group of ballet dancers. So even within a group of very flexible people, there are genetic differences that affect how flexible they can become, in spite of their physiques and hours of practice.[37]

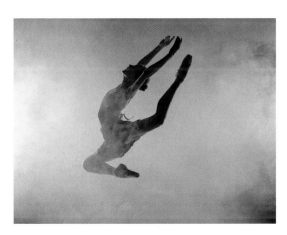

Figure 5.1 (a) Some people are naturally more flexible. Photograph courtesy of Shutterstock.

37 Kim et al., 2014.

It has also been shown that levels of flexibility are similar in family members even after 7 years.[38] So if you feel that you are "naturally inflexible," there may be a genetic basis for that.

Interestingly, our flexibility in different movements is also influenced by genetics to differing degrees. A twin study (identical and non-identical) that focused on the lower back showed that flexibility in leaning forward was more related to genetics than flexibility in leaning back, which was more influenced by lifestyle and physical habits.[39] This may mean that some of your tight areas are caused more by your genes and others more by your lifestyle. Why not ask your family members if they are tight in the same area, especially if you have a twin.

It is interesting to note that our fascia, which is such a key aspect of our flexibility, also displays genetic differences. There is a strong correlation between your level of genetically endowed strength and your flexibility. Stronger people have a tighter fascial net, which makes them less flexible, whereas lighter, slimmer people have looser fascia, allowing them greater flexibility.[40] The theory is that naturally stronger people have more fibroblasts, which therefore lay down more fascia, and more flexible people have fewer fibroblasts, and therefore less fascia.

However, even though our genes have set us up to be flexible, inflexible, hypermobile, tight, weaker or stronger, there is no reason that we cannot improve on what we have been given ourselves. Whatever our "genetic starting point" is, we can develop our bodies through the right kind of training and lifestyle, boosting our flexibility and strength. Or to paraphrase Dr Mehmet Oz: "Your genetics load the gun. Your lifestyle pulls the trigger."

Age

The differences between a baby, lying completely flat on her front with her legs and arms out to the side, and a 70-year-old who can barely look up are obviously huge. Babies are soft, relaxed and open, while older

people tend to be stiff, more closed-up in their posture, and have a smaller range of motion.

Aside from age-related changes, part of the reason for this is if that you do not use it, you do lose it, so a lot of stiffness in aging seems to be caused by people starting to act "like old people." Many people have the belief that the elderly cannot move and if they do they will injure themselves, so as they age they restrict themselves to smaller and smaller patterns of movement and are often rigid with fear when they do move—causing further tension and rigidity in their muscles and connective tissue.

Another aspect of increased inflexibility in older age is dehydration in the tissues, including the fascia (caused by reduced movement), which then stiffens, restricting movement even further.[41]

Many of my clients look more youthful since starting to stretch and I personally feel that resistance stretching has an anti-aging effect on the fascia and other tissues. Part of the mechanism is possibly through helping to re-hydrate it, as the movement combined with tension wrings the old fluid out of the tissue and when it is released, it "sucks up" fresh fluid. In addition there is strong evidence to show that stretching reduces inflammation[42] (chronic inflammation goes hand in hand with aging).

Therefore, although age is obviously a factor, since our bodies and quality of tissue do change over time, I would not entirely blame age for inflexibility; it is far more likely to be due to physical habits and lifestyle. In truth I have seen clients in their 20s, 30s and 60s with equal levels of flexibility, so I recommend that if you are a little younger, keep stretching and moving to prevent immobility later in life. And if you are a little older, you can use the stretching to increase mobility, but it is best to build up slowly, as you may need a little more recovery time than when you were 20.

38 Katzmarzyk et al., 2001. 39 Battié et al., 2008. 40 Myers, 2014.

41 Myers, 2012. 42 Berrueta et al., 2015.

> *"Age is an issue of mind over matter. If you don't mind, it doesn't matter."*
>
> *Mark Twain*

Movement Habits

Through our babyhood and infancy, our body develops its musculature and fascial system, allowing us to sit up, crawl, walk and eventually run and we naturally develop healthy restrictions in our fascia which keep our movements supported and our joints stable. Otherwise we would fall over all the time and our limbs would fly out in all directions. We need the structure of fascia to support clean, energy-efficient movements, helping to channel the force of our muscles. Over time our fascia becomes the documentary of our physical lives, almost completely shaped by it (as well as partly shaped by our genetic blueprint of course). For many of us that looks like hours spent sitting in chairs and sofas, as well as mainly forward-orientated, rather than side-to-side, horizontal or backward, movements, as well as hours hunched over books and screens. Although it may not seem like sitting would do us much damage, it can actually lead to more connective tissue building up, which can restrict us like scar tissue does.[43]

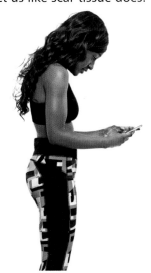

Figure 5.2 Our day-to-day posture has a huge impact on the condition and shape of our fascia.

Most of us do not realize just how much our social norms shape our bodies, through limiting which movements are socially acceptable. In reality the way we walk, sit, dance, and how often we do these things, is extremely proscribed, and to go against these rules is to risk social exclusion or even be thought insane! The sight of a small child running wildly, arms flailing, may be funny and even inspirational to us, but the sight of a businessman doing the same thing is worrying, even frightening. However, I have put some tips on increasing your variety of movement below, under Tips for the Naturally Inflexible.

Gender

It is widely believed that women are more flexible than men and there is some scientific evidence to support this. Part of the reason is thought to be that women's wider pelvises allow a greater range of motion of the hips than men's narrower pelvises do. But more importantly, hormones have a sizeable impact on flexibility in women as, during the phase of the menstrual cycle where estrogen and relaxin are highest, collagen production decreases by 40%.[44] As mentioned before, lower collagen production is linked to higher levels of flexibility. However, there are some differences among studies as to which point in the cycle has the higher risk, some finding a higher risk at the beginning[45] and others during ovulation.[46] These studies also show a reduction in ACL strength in women when estrogen and relaxin are at higher levels. This suggests that women who are about to participate in sports where the risk of ACL tear is higher should probably not stretch straight beforehand.

In my own practice I have seen that women do tend to be more flexible than men, but I have seen a huge variation between individuals within each gender. The long and short of this is that when it comes to resistance stretching, it does not matter what gender you are, it only matters that you do what you have to do (if anything) to become more balanced.

34 Bowman, 2014. 44 Silvers and Mandelbaum, 2007. 45 Slauterbeck et al., 2002. 46 Wojtys et al., 1998.

Diet and Flexibility

The connection between fascia and diet is not something that has been researched exhaustively, but there is evidence that the pH of your tissue (acid or alkaline) has an influence on the health of your tissue including your fascia, as it affects all of the biochemical reactions in the body. In the body, pH influences how much oxygen our tissue uses, how our blood clots, and how well our immune system works.[47] Acidity can increase how much the edges of a wound contract (by increasing the amount that the cells with this function, named myofibroblasts, contract) so it is possible that acidity may affect the tension of the fascia.[48] In addition, people with lower back pain who took an alkaline nutritional supplement for a month said that their pain had halved, so it is possible that an alkaline pH may benefit the fascia in some people.[49]

Another way that pH affects our fascial health concerns the lubrication that oils our machine. The deep fascia secretes hyaluronic acid to lubricate and aid sliding between it and the epimysium (fibrous tissue covering) of the muscle it is lying against. However, this lubrication can go the other way and become an adhesive glue when our tissue is overused, underused or even if we get stressed. This stickiness can be reduced by a more alkaline environment.[50]

A more alkaline diet is said to lower the acidity of the body, by removing acidity-causing foods (for example, although lemon is acidic, it has an alkaline effect in the body). There isn't a large amount of scientific data to back this up, but since the diet is basically full of fresh fruit and vegetables, is low on carbs and salt, and includes absolutely no processed foods, it is likely to provide a health benefit for many people, especially for those with an unhealthy diet.

However, I am not a nutritionist and I have seen different types of diet work for different people, therefore I would not recommend any one particular diet for everyone. I would suggest that you find what works best for you, perhaps by going to see a qualified nutritionist.

Physical Health

Many chronic health conditions impact the fascia. For example, in some stroke or spinal cord injury patients the fascia can stiffen so much that surgery may be required to relieve the tension. Or, as mentioned in Chapter 2, in Dupuytren's contracture the fascia of the palm can thicken and tighten, greatly restricting movement in the hand.

Because the fascia is a body-wide network, it makes sense that it is affected by, or may even partly be the cause of, systemic health issues. (**Caution**: If you do have an issue like this, make sure that you ask your doctor before starting to stretch to make sure resistance stretching is appropriate. Also I recommend that if you do stretch, take it nice and slowly and do not only focus on the problem area).

Traumatic injury to the body, such as in an accident, causes the fascia to build in that area and any other area affected, in order to stabilize the body. Even accidents that we think are minor or happened too long ago to affect us may be impacting the structure and biomechanics of our body, due to the long-lasting built-up fascia. If you have been knocked out of balance at any time, you may need to stretch through some old, thickened fascia to right yourself again.

Emotional Health

It might sound a bit airy-fairy, but of course your emotions affect your body; just look at someone who is obviously feeling a specific emotion—they usually have the posture and physiology to match. For example, an angry person often has a tense, almost rigid body, ready for fight or flight (usually in terms of their state, rather than actually going to fight or run away), a red face and shallow or held breath. A happy person usually breathes more slowly and deeply, moves more freely and easily, and is more open and upright in their posture, looking up more often than down.

47 Klingler, 2015. 48 Pipelzadeh & Naylor, 1998. 49 Vormann et al., 2001. 50 Muscolino, 2012.

It has already been proven that emotion has a huge impact on physiology and health as well as the way we hold ourselves, and I believe it also has an impact on our fascia. If that emotional state is anger, feeling down, hopeless, or unmotivated it will likely have a detrimental effect on their flexibility. On the other hand, I would expect that happiness, optimism, excitement and other positive feelings would make one more flexible.

There is evidence to show that yoga can help us to relax, having a positive effect on our physiology, including breathing, blood circulation, and blood pressure.[51] So, although emotions can create an unhealthy physical state, we can change that physical state through stretching. This means that we can improve our emotions by using stretching to alter our physical state. Or in other words, feeling better can probably help to keep you more flexible and you can also stretch to feel better.

> *"Most psychologists treat the mind as disembodied, a phenomenon with little or no connection to the physical body. Conversely, physicians treat the body with no regard to the mind or the emotions. But the body and mind are not separate, and we cannot treat one without the other."*
>
> *Candace Pert*

So, now that we have discussed most of the reasons that someone may be naturally more or less flexible, it is important to say that it does not really matter which you are; it is just helpful to understand your starting point, and what you can do to help yourself.

Broadly speaking, naturally flexible people need to strengthen themselves more and naturally inflexible people need to stretch themselves more. However, even people who are very flexible have certain areas that are tight and need to be worked on, while even very strong people have areas that are very weak. Luckily resistance stretching both strengthens and stretches you, so you can work on improving yourself through a balanced and consistent resistance stretching practice.

Extra Tips on Boosting ROM through Movement for the "Naturally Inflexible"

> *"Our strength grows out of our weakness."*
>
> *Ralph Waldo Emerson*

If you are not "naturally flexible," it is tempting to stick to your strengths and avoid stretching at all costs. You actually need the opposite—a regular stretching practice starting at a level that is suitable for you and increasing slowly and sustainably. Try not to focus on how inflexible you are, as if it is a problem. Focus on what you notice and feel whilst stretching and enjoying the benefits as they come.

It is also sensible to make sure that you are moving through a range of varying movements every day, whether through planned exercise, or just moving. Here are some tips for the "naturally stiff" to help you become more flexible:

1. *Sit on the floor at home*, while you are watching the TV, reading a book or with family and friends. Whilst you are on the floor sit in a variety of ways and move around from time to time. You can squat, sit with legs crossed, out in front of you, out in a V shape in front of you, with one knee bent in front of you and the other up, or with legs bent (one in front and one behind).

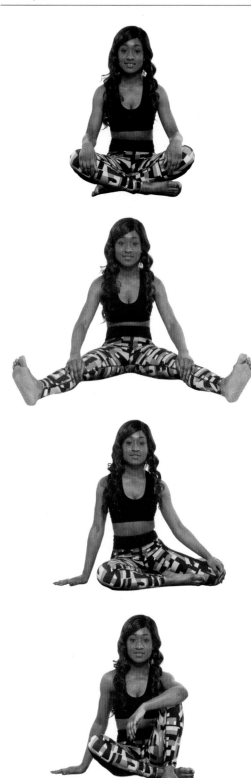

This may be uncomfortable at first, but persist (unless you have a medical or physical issue that it aggravates) and it will get easier, and you will find that your hips become looser and that it is easier to move.

2. *Stretch the way your body is telling you to*. When you are quite mindful of your body, you will notice that when you have been still for a while, your body feels a certain way. It might feel like a lack of sensation, or a kind of boredom of the body. This is the body's way of saying it would like you to move and get some more blood and fluid circulating. Usually, if you do move, your body starts to feel more zingy and alive—this is the way bodies are meant to feel most of the time.

3. *Slowly start to increase your range of movement*, with a gentle and patient attitude. You can do this in many ways; for example, while walking you could increase your stride length for a few steps at a time to stretch your hips a little. Consciously exaggerate some of the movements that you make throughout the day (but not all of them), so that you end up moving outside your normal range of motion. But do not push yourself hard, or through pain at all. This should be an easy, enjoyable thing to do.

Most of us are as flexible as the movements we make on a daily basis. Therefore, part of the solution to greater flexibility is simply to move more. Simple really! Increased movement is very important in helping to re-pattern, in effect "re-train" our fascia. If you are chronically inflexible then increasing your range of movement, and the range of movements you make, will support the improvements in your stretching enormously. Resistance stretching can especially help to work through the excess fascia that has built up over years, which is often very tough and dense.

Figure 5.3 Ways to sit at home.

I am not suggesting that we move like nobody is watching, because, well, people often *are* watching. However, you can try being mindful of the movements you always make and then (when the coast is clear, or you are somewhere where you feel you can move freely) start trying to make all the movements you do not normally make. Moving sideways or diagonally, squatting, crawling, reaching in all different directions, jumping. And even though these movements may feel unnatural to you at first, due to your built-up fascia and the surprise of your un-prepared muscles, over time your body will catch on. You do not need to run like a crazy person but do try to increase what is on your menu, movement-wise.

4. *Do not binge-stretch*. After decades of use our fascia has learned what we like to do and supports us in those movements, so that infrequent bursts of exercise, sporadic yoga classes, or sudden unfamiliar movements, for example, can be surprising to the body and painful. Therefore, do not try to make up for a lifetime's lack of stretching by doing it all at once! By easing into it you will get your body on board, rather than fighting it. Actually, strangely, "fighting the stiffness" is a common attitude I have seen in people who are naturally less flexible. I am not sure why, but they often seem to have a more goal-oriented outlook that sees parts of their bodies as problems to be solved. Bodies do not like this and more often than not, will stiffen up even more as a result.

Extra Tips on Boosting Strength Through Resistance Stretching for the "Naturally Less Strong"

I didn't want you to feel left out! Although you may be wonderfully flexible in many ways, do you feel that you could be a little stronger? Well, resistance stretching can actually strengthen you also. Because we tense the muscles and move, it makes each stretch an eccentric strength movement also.

Rather than giving you tips for your daily life, I would like to give you some specific tips for your stretching that I have found useful for those who could use a bit more strength.

1. *Do not avoid your weak areas*. Our bodies are masters of using the very strongest bits of ourselves to make a movement, because that is the most logical and efficient way to do it. I often see clients who have very weak areas that started off a little weaker, resulting in the body avoiding using them so they became weaker still. This is a bit like never wanting to work with the inexperienced person in your office, so they never gain experience and fall even further behind. Therefore, when you are stretching and a certain part is difficult (but not painful, and you are within your ROM), keep going through it rather than around it. This takes some mental focus as it is so natural to us to avoid these areas. Then when we do go through them it feels a bit rubbish sometimes, not painful, just a bit "ughhh." On the same note, do not avoid any specific stretches that are harder because you feel weak doing them.

2. *Build up slowly*. As this form of stretching is strengthening also, it is like a workout and you can get a bit of muscle ache afterwards. Do not put yourself off for life by majorly overdoing it and then thinking it is an awful thing to do to yourself. It is only sore because you really need to do it. The only way beyond that is to go through it, but at a reasonable pace and with rest days in between when you first start.

3. *Drink plenty of water*. If you are working your muscles more than you are used to you will also have more of the by-products of muscle use than you are used to, so flush those out by drinking sufficient water (a maximum of 2 L in a day is enough for most people). This will also help with the stiffness and also to re-hydrate your tissue on your rest days.

4. *Be patient*. Strength is not built in a day. Just keep stretching on a regular basis and you will start to see good improvements over time. But you cannot rush this. If you would like to measure the improvement, why not try a classic exercise, such as a push-up, before you start stretching and then see how much easier they get as you continue on your stretching journey.

5. *Add some strength workouts*. If you have access to a gym and/or personal trainer then the stretching will fit in quite neatly to your workouts. If you do not have access to either of these things, then you can do bodyweight exercises at home, using a book or an app. Just make sure you follow the instructions carefully to avoid injury. Just do your stretching between workout days, or after your workouts, as long as you are not too tired!

So whether you are naturally stronger or more flexible, resistance stretching has some tools to help uncover your physical potential. Apart from the clear benefit to your body, this can make a big difference to the rest of your life as well.

> *"Flexibility helps you to adapt to the world and all the s**t that comes your way. Strength gives you the resilience to stand your ground and stand up for what you believe in.*
>
> *A strong and flexible body = a force to be reckoned with."*
>
> Suzanne Wylde

The Benefits of a Regular Stretching Practice

Can you imagine being on the bus, the train, the street, in a coffee shop or your workplace, surrounded by people with strong, functional, healthy and happy bodies? Can you see how happy, independent, interesting, motivated, helpful, empowered, and imaginative they are? How good they are to work with, fun to be around, and easy to talk to? Can you visualize a class or a school bus full of children who are responsive, easy and spontaneous in their movements, balanced and open in their posture, who bear no sign of hunching over desks or technology for hours, and are just as happy swinging in a tree as sitting on a sofa? Watch how their bodies are not distorted from being confined over the years to a chair at home, at school, at work, or on holiday and finally in retirement homes, as they mature and age. Can you see a future for yourself where instead of inevitably slowing, shrinking, and breaking down, you open up, grow stronger, taller, healthier, more flexible and agile?

Stretching is not a miracle drug that magically gives you special powers. Or is it? With strengthening, stretching, anti-aging, and posture-boosting properties, resistance stretching might just be that secret weapon you need in order to be the best you can be. Of course, stretching by itself is not enough. You still need to eat good food, drink enough water, sleep enough, exercise, socialize and have fun to be healthy. But by stretching your fascia, you can strip away the layers of inactivity, poor posture, sitting, stress, and tension, revealing your true wonderful self. I have seen amazing changes in my clients and this book contains all the information you need to do the same.

What Stretching Can Do For Us

In case that is not enough reason to stretch, I have listed some of the main benefits of stretching below. Please note, that where the points I make are supported by research the study is listed, and that some of these benefits are exclusive to resistance stretching, whereas others apply to other stretching and movement techniques also.

1. It Promotes the Flow of Blood and Fluid in our Bodies

Because we are designed to move, some of our bodily functions only work well with movement (which in previous generations was more of a "given"). For example, the calf muscles are designed to help blood return from the lower legs to the heart, but if we are not using them by walking around then they will not be able to do this as well. This effect is compounded by the fact that chronically tight muscles reduce circulation even further, leading to some tissue that is less hydrated and well fed (supplied with nutrients). Therefore the movement aspect of the stretching helps to improve blood and fluid circulation.

2. It Can Help with Specific Physical Issues

Many of us have been to a physiotherapist, or other type of therapist, and been given stretching exercises to do. It is clear that in order to have a well-balanced and functioning body, we need to have flexible and strong muscles, and that tension in specific areas can cause problems in alignment, function and even pain. For example, stretching can help greatly in cases of long-term lower back pain.[52]

3. It Helps to Prevent the Onset of Stiffness and Limited Movement

As we age we can stiffen up, experiencing smaller and smaller ranges of movement; we may find it harder to bend down, get up off the floor, and eventually even walk properly. Stretching helps us to stay strong and flexible, keeping our sphere of physical influence larger and preventing us from curling up like a frightened hedgehog.

4. It Reconditions and Re-Patterns Our Fascia

I speak more about this in the section on Resistance Stretching and the Fascia (Chapter 3), but I believe that resistance stretching can move us out of the fascial ruts we create in our bodies by using them in the same ways over and over again, freeing us from these restrictions. The resistance also lets us work through the stuck and older bits of our fascia, freshening and rejuvenating it.

5. It Can Boost our Mood

Stretching can reduce stress, whilst strength training can boost self-esteem, reduce anxiety, and improve mental functioning.[53] Although there have been no studies on the specific effects of resistance stretching on mood, I have seen my students growing in confidence, optimism, mental adaptability, and resilience.

Posture has also been shown to have an enormous impact on our psychological state.

One study showed that hunching forward often leads to depression, a feeling of hopelessness and powerlessness, and brings up negative memories. This is scary because almost everyone spends time hunched over! Skipping, however, was shown to reverse the damage.[54] The posture we adopt has even been shown to affect how confident we are about our own thoughts.[55]

My clients often appear to have increased confidence and positivity, and report feeling more energetic. No one has ever come with the express purpose (that they have told me) of improving their mood and energy levels, but I have yet to see anyone who did not look happier and more confident from regular resistance stretching.

6. It Improves our Performance

Many of us think that stretching will help us somehow; in our lives, our sport, our posture, or elsewhere, but we may not put our finger on exactly how. Well, a study on the effect of regular stretching (40 minutes three times a week, for 10 weeks) found that it improved, not only people's flexibility, but their strength, sprinting speed, and power output also.[56] This is at odds with recent research suggesting that stretching decreases performance in sprinters (more on that in Chapter 9). Most of the benefits were thought to have been the result of increased strength, bringing us to the next point.

7. Stretching Can Make you Stronger

Most of us think about hitting the weights when we want to become stronger, but we do not think about having a good stretch. According to a study, muscles become significantly stronger after stretching, possibly due to an increase in myoblasts (cells that can become muscle cells),[57] but also due to the fact that we can remove fascia that may be restricting muscle growth. I talk about why bodybuilders are resistance stretching to improve their gains in Resistance Stretching and the Fascia (Chapter 3).

52 Sherman et al., 2011. 53 Steckl, 2014.

54 Peper & Lin, 2012. 55 Brinol et al., 2009.
56 Kokonnen et al., 2007. 57 Day et al., 1997.

8. Health

It seems incredible, but the flexibility of your hamstrings is linked to the flexibility of your arteries. Researchers found that people who did badly on the sit and reach test also had stiffer arteries, making them more vulnerable to stroke and heart disease.[58] If that news does not make you want to stretch I don't know what will!

Also, hypermobility, which is often thought of as "too much flexibility," is linked to lower rates of osteoarthritis in the knees and better bone density in the hips (at around 55 years of age)[59] so there may be a connection between flexibility and improved joint health, especially as we age. Which brings us nicely to the next point.

9. Anti-aging

Over the years of teaching stretching and stretching people, I have seen wonderful improvements in people's faces and bodies, which make it look like the tension, tiredness, stress and, yes, even age are being stripped away. One study showed that older people who stretched for 4 weeks had a walking gait similar to that of young people.[60] This is great, not only because it shows that stretching can reverse some of what we think of as the "unavoidable" consequences of aging, but it shows that you can start to improve your physical condition at almost any age.

10. Stretching Helps to Release Emotions and Trauma

Stretching the fascia is amazing for releasing pent-up emotions as well as trauma from the body. If you are not aware of having any, then this part may be hard to relate to, but if you have experienced trauma to your body (whether from an accident or violence), or have had a tough time emotionally and are still feeling "not quite right" or "not yourself," I believe that you will know what I am talking about. In many ways the body is an extension of the unconscious mind and many things we cannot deal with (such as shock, anger, or another emotion) at the time get stored in our bodies, expressing themselves as pain, tension, thickening, immobility, protective postures and more.

Luckily, we do not need to know exactly what to work on, we just need to start stretching ourselves and see what comes up. For the most part things will only come out if we are ready to deal with them, yet I still recommend that you have a trained therapist or counselor in reserve that you can go to in case you feel overwhelmed or in need of support.

I have had clients who have experienced accidents and whose bodies still feel as though they are in the protective holding pattern that was created (with the fascia) at the time of the accident. If you feel that this applies to you, know that the body needs to feel safe in order to unwind, so pushing yourself hard is really not going to help. Go gently and slowly and work your way in over time. Do not be surprised if some of the shock and other emotions that you could not handle at the time of the accident come up to be processed and released. The best attitude to have is non-judgment and lots of self-compassion and it is best to be in private, or with a trained therapist (from talking/alternative/movement-based techniques is probably best). Breathing will help you to move these emotions through, just follow your body's feeling of how it wants to breathe and let go, rather than adhering to any breathing protocols.

This may all seem rather too deep for a stretching book to those who are not aware of any emotions stuck in their body and who are lucky enough not to have suffered any trauma. If you were to tell me there is nothing emotional about your body, it just needs to be stretched, I would say that you would be the first person like that I have met. Having said that, it is completely fine to focus on the physical side of the stretching as, if

58 Yamamoto et al., 2009. 59 Dolan et al., 2002. 60 Cristopoliski et al., 2009.

anything aside from that needs to happen, it will happen naturally. For some people the stretching is purely physical, and for others it is not. It is what you make it at the end of the day, and what you need from your stretching will likely change from week to week and over the years.

You may have initially thought that you needed to stretch because your flexibility needs work, but looking at how many other benefits there are to stretching, how could you afford not to? I do not want to sound like the typical specialist and say it is all about one thing, that is, stretching, but with all the improvements that I have observed in my clients over the years, I can safely say that it is one of the most transformative things you can do, and resistance stretching in particular. Becoming happier, healthier, better at your sport, younger, and emotionally more free. Who could ask for more than that?

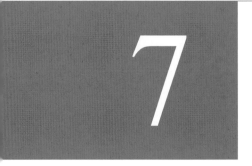

7 Resistance Stretching FAQs

Here are some of the questions beginners most commonly ask.

1. How is this different to "normal" (static) stretching?

In static stretching you try to become more flexible by pushing beyond your current ROM, while in resistance stretching you only move within your natural ROM. Unlike static stretching, it also strengthens the muscles.

2. Is it like yoga or Pilates?

Resistance stretching is not about holding certain poses as is common in yoga, but moving almost continuously, whilst maintaining tension in the muscles throughout that movement. And whereas Pilates mainly focuses on strengthening the core and increasing stability through fairly gentle and controlled movements, resistance stretches are more challenging and focus more removing tension and adhesions in the fascia.

3. How is resistance stretching different to using resistance bands?

We do not use resistance bands in resistance stretching. The only thing they have in common is that both can strengthen you, but the movements are very different and you cannot use a resistance band for resistance stretching as they are too stretchy to be able to move you against resistance.

4. I am very inflexible, will I be able to do it?

Yes, because the stretching is self-tailoring. If you can only move a small distance in a stretch, then you do that. Do that movement with resistance repeatedly and it will slowly (or sometimes quickly) improve.

5. I am not very strong, can I do it?

Yes, and doing it will make you stronger. Tense your muscles to around 70% of your ability and do as many repetitions as you can comfortably manage (up to the recommended amount) and you will start to strengthen your muscles. You should notice a difference in only days or weeks.

6. Should I be sore after the stretching?

I find that roughly one fifth of people who are new to resistance stretching feel a little sore afterwards, and it seems to be dependent on their unique physiology as well as their current level of exercise/activity. Generally the better conditioned your body, the less likely you are to be sore. Any soreness is likely to be a result of the strength component of the stretching; it is like a post-workout muscle ache. Just keep moving, drinking enough water, and maybe try a sea salt bath.

7. Should it hurt when I stretch, as in no-pain, no-gain?

No, it should never hurt when you stretch. We are not looking to push through any pain at all, though discomfort is sometimes acceptable.

8. Can I do it if I'm in pain?

It is best to consult with a doctor or physiotherapist before stretching if you have been injured or are in pain. Also, if you are already in pain and have been for a while, then it is best not to directly stretch the painful area and not to stretch if it increases your level of pain. I have put some more guidelines on this in the How to Stretch section (Chapter 9).

9. How often should I stretch?

I recommend that when you start you should stretch at least three times a week. I have put some guidelines on how often to stretch in the How to Stretch section (Chapter 9).

10. How long will I keep the changes?

If you stretch only once then you will probably lose all or most of the changes after a few days or a week. If you stretch regularly, you will keep more of a change. If you stretch regularly for a sustained period, say 4 weeks, 2 months, or longer, you may be able to bring about positive changes that you do not lose. As long as you are not causing the issue again through poor posture or other habits, you can change your fascia for the better and not revert to your former state.

11. Should I stretch before exercise?

This is a bit controversial. Generally speaking, I would say that if you are "naturally inflexible" it does help to stretch before exercise, after warming up for 5–10 minutes. But if you are doing any sports that require a lot of efficiency, such as sprinting, and you are new to resistance stretching it is best not to stretch in the 40 minutes right before you train/compete to be on the safe side. In that case you can stretch later in the day, and still feel the benefit to your biomechanics, movement, and performance.

12. Can I stretch whilst I have an injury? Will it help me to recover?

Often you can stretch, as long as your doctor or physio says it is OK. I recommend staying away from the injured area, stretching around it, and further away. This often helps by relieving the tension on the area. Stretching has also been shown to reduce inflammation, which should help. However, I do not recommend directly stretching a recently injured area.

13. I've just had surgery, should I stretch?

It is best to wait for 6 weeks or so. Because the fascia is all connected, you may inadvertently pull on the part of you that is trying to heal. After this time, if it has healed completely, you can start stretching, which may help to remove unwanted scar tissue. But ease into stretching, do not overdo it!

14. How can I make a stretch stronger?

If you tense more, then you will be resisting more and that makes the stretch more powerful. The downside is that you can ache more afterwards, especially if you are not properly warmed up! So only tense more if you are warmed up and not in pain or injured.

15. Does creating tension in muscles in order to resistance stretch ever make muscles more tense?

It can do if you tense muscles that are in pain or have been tense for a long time. I recommend trying to stretch them gently and if they do not respond by feeling more relaxed, then avoid them completely and do not tense them while you stretch other areas. This does take a bit of focus as many of us tense our tight muscles automatically.

16. Why is resistance stretching good/important for me?

It is good for you because it is a healthy, whole-body, and natural way to stretch and strengthen your body. It helps to flush toxins out of your tissues, to strengthen you where you are weak, and to release you where you are tight.

17. What is fascia? Why is it important for me/ my health to consider the fascia?

Fascia is the dense connective tissue that runs from your head to your toes and all around your body, making you the shape that you are. Because it can either support you in good posture and healthy movements or hold you down into poor posture and restrict your movements, it is very important that it is in good condition.

18. How can you determine the "health" of the fascia and whether it needs to be stretched or not?

I can tell when I do walking massage on people, when I stretch them, or when I feel their tissue (by gently squeezing their arm, for example because I have a fair bit of experience in working with people and their bodies). If you are new to stretching you may only be able to feel that your fascia is restricted in some places, but it is unusual to be aware of the state of your fascia until you are a bit more experienced. The best way to feel the difference between obviously tight and obviously unrestrictive fascia is to do two or three stretches on one side of the body only and then walk around, so that you can compare the feeling in each side. More experienced people often sense the quality of their fascia through the sensations in their bodies when they move.

19. What kind of problems can resistance stretching be especially helpful for?

Resistance stretching is great for poor posture, lack of strength, restricted movement, general lack of energy and "go," improving biomechanics, and boosting performance and it can also increase dexterity, grace, and precision of movements.

20. What does the science or research say about resistance stretching?

Not very much research has been done yet on resistance stretching, but Professor Guimberteau has found that resistance stretching helps to align the fibers within the fascia. The science supports different aspects of resistance stretching, with positive effects shown from stretching in general, eccentric training, and movement.

21. How can resistance stretching be used with other forms of exercise or treatments?

Resistance stretching plays very well with others, so you can fit it in with most other exercise routines. Generally speaking I would say if you are about to do something that requires more flexibility then stretching beforehand is great. If you are about to do something requiring a lot of efficiency such as sprinting or long jump, then it is best to stretch afterwards or later in the day. For regular gym goers, stretching at the end of a workout works very well.

If you are about to go for osteopathy, physiotherapy, or chiropractic, I would not stretch beforehand on the same day unless they say that you can (your increased flexibility may have an impact on their diagnosis and the effect of their treatment). It is fine to stretch before massage or other alternative therapies.

22. Is it possible to injure myself with resistance stretching?

Yes, as it is possible to injure yourself with almost any exercise or stretching technique. Therefore it is important that you get medical advice first if you need to, follow the guidelines in the How to Stretch section (Chapter 9), and always stay within your natural range of motion and do not try to push beyond that. Also, make sure that you are warmed up and do not overdo the stretching when you start, even if you are excited.

Most commonly people just feel a bit achy after their first few sessions and this eases off. This is especially true of those who need a lot more strength, those who are very "naturally inflexible," or those who do not do any form of exercise at all. If you are in any of those categories, just keep going as long as you are only experiencing muscle ache rather than real pain. Your body will adapt.

23. Can I combine resistance stretching with other forms of stretching to get more of a benefit?

If you have already been doing the other form of stretching for a while and are experienced and without any injuries, I would say that it would be fine to add a couple of Moving Stretches in. It is important that you do not overdo it, for example, if you already stretch for an hour every day, and add another hour of resistance stretching. People who are safer mixing types of stretching include dancers and athletes as they have usually already been stretching for a long time and know what works for their bodies. However, even if you are experienced, resistance stretching is a bit of a stronger technique, so please just try a few stretches at one time, if adding them to an already rigorous routine.

24. How long do I need to keep stretching for?

Many people experience a lot of change right away, then often plateau for a while, and then break through to a new level of benefits, including more youthful looks and much better posture. So if you hold on and stretch for the long-term you may get even better results than you expect.

25. How soon will I feel the benefits of resistance stretching?

About 99% of students feel amazing after their first class, so I would say right away. You may not get the exact benefit that you want right away, but it is likely that you will feel freer, taller, more open, energized, and lighter. So get stretching!

8 Flexibility Questionnaires

Tracking your flexibility is an essential tool in understanding the state of your body and in deciding how to progress with your stretching. It can help to show you; where you lack flexibility, how you are progressing and how stretching is benefitting you. It can even give you a clue of what or what is and isn't working for you. If you also track your mental and emotional state you will have an even better idea of where you are and the wider improvements to your well-being that may occur.

In this section I have included these different ways of tracking your progress:

1. flexibility self-tests
2. health and flexibility questions
3. mood and energy questions
4. posture photographs
5. pose, stretch, or movement photographs and videos
6. keeping a stretching diary

In a sports lab they would have specialized equipment to measure your flexibility very precisely, but the basic tests in this section are great for giving you a rough idea of your flexibility level right now. I recommend that you at least do the self-tests and the questions; however, photographs give the most obvious evidence of changes in posture and a stretching diary is the best way to bring together many different aspects of your life and health, allowing you to identify relationships between them, for example, between your sports performance and particular stretches, or between your stretching and your energy levels.

Do these tests right before you begin your new stretching regime, and continue at regular intervals (once a week or once a month, for example) so that you can keep track of your progress. I know many people who wish they had done this before they started! If you decide to keep a stretching journal you can keep the results in that.

There are also some questions that will help you to record and track changes in your quality of life, covering any pain you are experiencing, health and energy levels. They are very subjective, of course, but can work well as a rough measure of your improvement. I recommend that when you re-do these tests and questions you start with a fresh page, so that you are not biased by looking at your previous answers. Also, it is best to try and perform them at the same time of day, in similar clothing.

To do these you will need: a piece of paper and a pen or electrical device to make a note of the answers, a pencil and/or piece of Blu-Tack, a tape measure, or failing that, a piece of string or shoelace which you will need to measure with a ruler after each test. For the photos you will need a camera, smartphone, tablet or laptop. It may be worth creating a separate folder to keep your photos in and I would save each with the date and position or pose as their file name (e.g., 7/9/17-front, 7/9/17-touching-toes), for quick reference.

Flexibility Self-Tests

Read the instructions, and perform these tests as shown. Do them with some effort, but comfortably, as straining will give you a false result. Table 8.1 is an example of the type of template you could use if you want to record the results like this. It is a good idea to make a note of how easy or hard each exercise is, as well as any other information, for example; what is getting in the way of being able to do the exercise. Also, five out of the six exercises require you to measure each side separately.

Test (and area being measured)	Distance	Notes
Touching toes (hamstrings)		
Sideways straight leg raise (abductor and adductors)	Left: Right:	
Knee to chest (hip flexors)	Left: Right:	
Trunk twist (torso and shoulders)	Left: Right:	
Elbow pull-back (chest)	Left: Right:	
Back scratch (arms and shoulders)	Left arm on top: Right arm on top:	

Table 8.1 Template for flexibility self-test

Touching Toes

(Hamstrings)

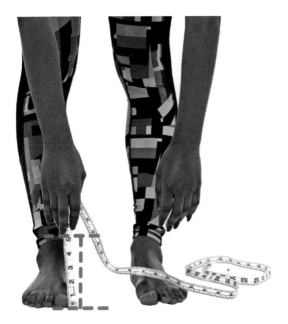

Standing with your feet close together and knees completely straight at all times, lean forward and touch your toes. If you cannot reach the ground, how many centimetres away are your fingertips? If you can put your hands on the ground then stand on a step and measure how many centimetres below your feet you can go. If your fingers are 5 cm above your toes, write the result as 5 cm above. If they are 5 cm below, write 5 cm below.

Sideways Straight Leg Raise

(Abductor and adductors)

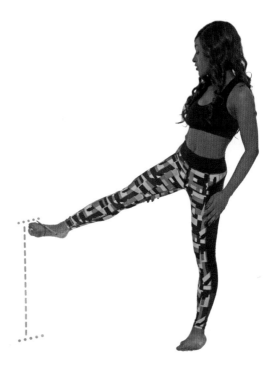

Stand straight and lift one leg out to the side. How far off the ground can you lift it? Please note that it is fine to hold onto something for support, but do not lean over with your torso. Do both sides recording the measurements separately.

This can be tricky to measure by yourself, so you can attach a pencil to the foot that is pointing out sideways with an elastic band and make a small mark on the wall when your foot is raised as high as it can go. Try to make sure that the pencil is sticking out to the side, rather than up or down. This measures the flexibility of the adductors and the strength of the abductors.

Knee to Chest

(Hip flexors)

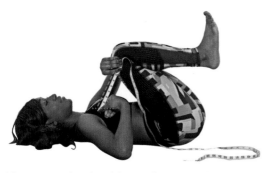

Lie on your back with one leg straight and one leg bent (the photo above should show one bent leg only). Pull your bent leg as close to your chest as is comfortable for you. Measure how far away your knee is from your chest using a tape measure or a piece of string.

Measure from the front side of your knees to your chest wall, rather than breasts or chest muscles, so that weight loss or gain does not impact the results. I recommend that you do this on both sides and record the results as 5 cm left, 6 cm right, for example, and if your knee is flat against your chest then record the result as 0.

Trunk Twist

(Torso and shoulders)

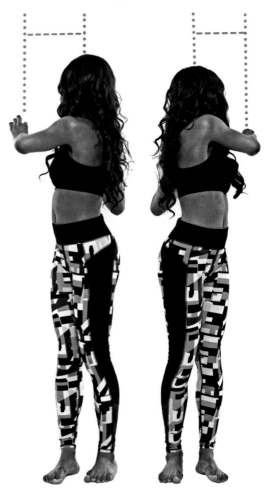

Draw a vertical line on a wall (or if you do not want to mark your wall, you can put a piece of Blu-Tack on it). Stand directly in front of this mark, facing away from the wall, an arm's length in front of it. With a piece of Blu-Tack in your right hand, twist to the right as far as you can reach comfortably and stick the Blu-Tack on the wall as a marker. Repeat this on the left and then measure both distances from the central mark.

Record the result of twisting towards the right, as the left side and vice versa for twisting to the left. If you managed to go beyond the central line, measure the result as "beyond" , e.g., 5 cm beyond.

Elbow Pull-Back

(Chest)

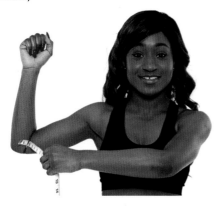

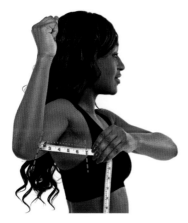

In a standing or sitting position, lift one arm up to your side, palm forward, with the elbow bent to 90° and level with the shoulder.

Pull your elbow backward as far as possible and measure how far back your elbow can go. Measure from the center of the side of your torso (so the center of your body as seen from the side).

This can be tricky to measure by yourself so you can put an elastic band around your elbow and put the tape measure into it, making a note of how much of it is sticking out. Draw your elbow back and then take the measurement from the center of your torso, deducting whatever length is sticking out the other side of the elastic band. For example if the reading at the center of the torso is 20 cm, but you have 10 cm of tape hanging out, then the actual measurement is 10 cm.

Back Scratch

(Arms and shoulders)

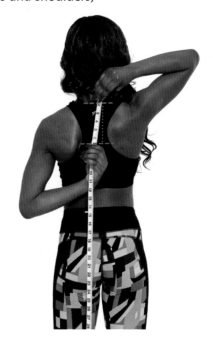

Stand comfortably and, reaching behind and up with one hand, and behind and down with the other, see how close you can bring your hands behind your back. If you cannot bring them together then record the distance. If you can overlap your hands, measure how far one hand can go beyond the other and record it as "beyond", e.g., 5 cm beyond.

If you are measuring this by yourself, then hold the beginning end of a tape measure or a piece of string in your upper hand and then grasp it as high up as you can with your bottom hand. Keep a hold of it with your bottom hand as you come out of the stretch and record the length. Try and hold the tape measure at a certain length in your upper hand so that you can deduct that afterwards (so if you are holding the tape measure at 3 cm with your upper hand and 10 cm at your lower hand, record the distance as 7 cm), thus making sure you have the exact measurement from fingertip to fingertip.

Health and Flexibility Questions

The questions listed below (in Table 8.2) are of course a little general and subjective, so please think about what you feel is true for you, on average. Please note that for the first two questions, 1 is poor and 10 is very good, whereas for the last two questions on limitation and pain, 10 is the worst and 0 is best. Of course it may seem silly to have a 0-rating, because then there is no issue to record. This is actually so that you will be able to keep an accurate record in the event that any of your issues resolve themselves completely.

Today's date:		
Question	**Answer**	**More info**
How would you rate your general health out of 10 (10 being the best, e.g., 6/10)?		
How would you rate your general flexibility on a scale 1–10 (10 being the best)?		
Does inflexibility currently limit you in any way, e.g., movement, exercise, performance or other? If so, please score each issue out of 10 (10 being the most problematic and 0 no issue at all)		
Do you have any main health/physical issues you hope the stretching will help? If so please rate the severity of the issue or pain level out of 10 (10 is the worst pain possible and 0 is no pain at all).		

Table 8.2 Health and flexibility questions

Mood and Energy Questions

These questions (in Table 8.3 below) are also a little general, so I recommend that you make a best guess based on your view of how you are day-to-day, rather than right this second. In terms of scoring, 1 is poor and 10 is very good, except for the appetite question at the end.

Today's date:		
Question	**Answer**	**More info**
Please rate your mood on a general day-to-day basis out of 10		
Please rate your energy levels on a day-to-day basis out of 10		
Please rate your sleep out of 10. For example, think about whether you get to sleep easily, your sleep is undisturbed, whether you wake up refreshed, etc.		
Please rate your appetite out of 10 (10 as the highest level of appetite)		

Table 8.3 Mood and energy questions

Posture Photographs

A great way of recording improvements in your posture as you stretch over time is to take a couple of photographs with your smartphone or camera before you get started and again at regular intervals, such as every week or 10 days. I recommend that you take your posture photos from three angles: facing toward the camera, sideways on, and facing away.

Here are some basic guidelines for taking your photos:

- Consistency is important so try to wear the same clothes, stand in the same place, with similar lighting, with or without shoes (without is better, but if you have to wear shoes for some reason, as long as this is the same in all photos it is fine), with a similar stance and from the same angle. This will make comparison much easier for you.

- It is important that the photo is straight, so that you can observe your posture more accurately. If you are taking a photo against a vertical line, such as a join in mirrors or a door frame, it is helpful to stand with the line directly through your midline so you can use it to see how symmetrical you are.

- It is great to take photos with yourself facing forward and side-on. You can also take a photo facing away. If you are by yourself you will have to use a timer or a mirror (the timer is preferable so that both of your arms can be down).

- Photos should be taken before you start and at fairly regular intervals—say once a week or once a month thereafter.

- Try to stand fairly naturally rather than sucking your tummy in or assuming an ideal posture. Stand with your feet hip-width apart and relaxed.

Changes that you may see in your photos include:

- improved posture
- better alignment of the body
- improved and more defined shape
- healthier coloring
- increased health and vitality
- more youthful looks

It can be hard to assess posture accurately without a lot of training, but you will likely be able to notice the above changes by yourself.

Forward-Facing Photograph

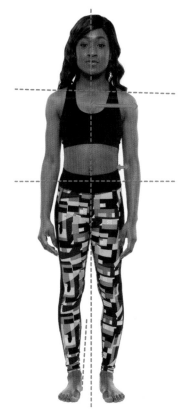

Draw a line through the center of the picture of your body, either on a computer or by holding a ruler or piece of string up to it. The line must be completely vertical, so start it in the center between the feet and draw it up from there in a straight line, regardless of where the head happens to be. *Notice*: Is your weight more on your right or left foot? Is your body roughly in line or do certain areas lean to one side more?

Then look at the following areas, observing key aspects:

1. Face: symmetry, health, shape?

2. Head: alignment above neck/ leaning toward one side?

3. Shoulders: raised or very close to midline of the body (it looks like they could be broader), is one higher than the other?

4. Neck: is it long or short looking?

5. Chest: open or closed (do the shoulders look like they are "looking inwardly", and so more closed, or "looking" forwards or outward and so more open)?

6. Arms: are the gaps between your arms and torso the same size on both sides?

7. Hands: are your palms facing backward, inward or forward?

8. Hips: are your "hip bones" (in common speech, i.e. where you "put your hands on your hips" not anatomical) even, or does one drop down?

9. Knees: do the centers of your kneecaps point in the same direction, and do you tend toward being "bow-legged" or "knock-kneed"?

10. Ankles: are your ankles collapsing inward at all, or fairly straight (look at your inner ankles)?

11. Are your feet pointing in the same direction?

Sideways Photograph

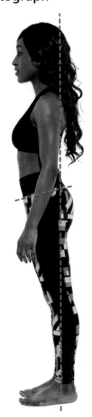

Stand sideways to the camera and try to remember to face the same way in each subsequent photograph.

Draw a line through the center of the side of your body from top to bottom. This line should be completely vertical and start in front of your ankle bone.

Is your ear, shoulder, hip bone, knee, and ankle roughly all in one line? Here are a few things to look for in your posture when you are standing side-on:

1. Head: does your head thrust forward, is it tipped forward (looking downward), or is it straight?

2. Shoulders: are they hunched forward, raised up toward the ears, or down and relaxed?

3. Upper back: is it hunched forward, or fairly straight?

4. Hips: are they flexed (with your bottom sticking out) or extended (with your bottom tucked in)?

Facing Away Photograph

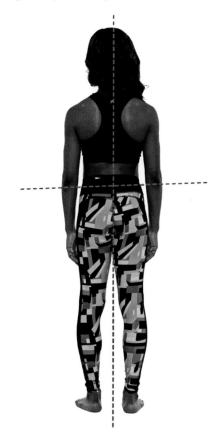

This may not seem like it would be very enlightening, but it can give you a great idea of the alignment in your spine, head, and hips. I recommend that you do it without a top on (a sports bra is fine) so that you can see the features of your back clearly.

Start the line in the center between the feet and draw it straight up from there. If you can see them, put a dot on the inside edge and upper edge of your shoulder blades.

1. Head: is it tilted to the side or straight?

2. Spine: is it completely straight?

3. Shoulder blades: is one closer to the spine than the other, is one higher than the other, or are they even?

4. Arms: look at the gap between your torso and your arms; is the gap even on both sides?

5. Hips: look for the top of your "hip bones;" are they level?

6. Achilles: look at the angle of the Achilles tendon on the back of your ankle; is it roughly vertical or does it bend?

By now, you have probably noticed some imperfections in your posture, which identifies you as an individual! Do not worry about this (unless you have a specific issue and then I recommend that you see a doctor, physio or osteopath, for example) as many people are a little out of balance. Even if you do have an issue and a postural imbalance, they may not be linked, just coincidental. If you feel that you require an exact postural assessment you will require the services of a professional.

From the first moment a pen was put into one of our hands and not the other we began our journey of biomechanical wonkiness, but many people function very well even so. In an ideal world we would be ambidextrous at everything; however, certain sports require a specific alignment for efficiency and power, so if you are functioning well and not in any pain then your posture may be perfect for what you are doing.

The purpose of keeping track of your posture is to see how it changes, and probably improves, through stretching. I have never seen it worsen in a client who was stretching regularly; however, I have seen existing underlying problems become exposed as substitutions (like cheating, but for the body) get stretched out. For example, if your posture generally improves, but the bottom of your ribs suddenly sticks out in front of you, for example, it could be due to the fact that your shoulders are no longer hunching forward and hiding the misalignment of your ribcage, which was there all along. You do not need to worry about the specifics unless you are a trained health or exercise professional, but any healthcare or physical therapist may be interested in seeing your photos if you go for a session, especially if you are seeking advice on a specific issue.

(As an aside, I highly recommend having a notebook just for your health and fitness, where you can record diagnoses, advice, and homework. Before you go for a session you can write down specific questions you want answered, as it is so easy to forget everything you wanted to know, and forget their advice and diagnosis too! It may also be useful for subsequent visits to other professionals.)

Pose, Stretch, and Movement Photographs and Videos

This is a great way to measure your progress toward specific goals if you are trying to improve in a dance or exercise movement, yoga pose, or a traditional stretch that you feel could be better.

For a pose or stretch you may find that a photo is better and taking video works best for recording the quality and range of a movement. You might want to take your photos and video from a couple of angles, to get the best sense of it.

Here are some guidelines for taking the best and most useful photos.

- Consistency is important. You need to do exactly the same movement/pose/stretch each time, of course, in shoes or not, and at a similar time of day is best. To make comparisons as easy as possible it is best to wear the same clothes, keep the location the same or similar, and have the same lighting.

- You may want to use a timer so that you have time to get into the correct position.

- Try to do the pose, stretch, or movement as best and as naturally as you can every time. There is no point in doing "before and after" photos if you are sucking in your tummy or smiling in the "after" photos, they should be done naturally so you can see the real results. The before and after photos later in this book were all done without any extra effort on the part of the models.

Changes that you may see in poses and stretches include:

- improved posture
- increased range of motion
- better alignment of the body
- more balanced left and right
- a more comfortable look.

Changes that you may see in movements include:

- improved posture
- greater dexterity and more nuanced subtle and fine movements
- improved co-ordination
- more strength
- better balance and poise
- greater range of motion
- smoother movements
- more grace and efficiency.

The interesting thing about improvements from your stretching is that although you can generally expect to have better posture, look taller and more open, move better and more gracefully and look more toned and integrated, you will also often get some surprising benefits that you did not expect. Each body is unique and has its own path to strength and flexibility.

Keeping a Stretching Diary

This is your personal diary, therefore you can keep track of whatever you like, depending on what you want to get out of the stretching. For example, if you want to improve your posture through stretching to improve your mood, confidence, and energy levels, I recommend that you make a note of each of these things alongside each stretching session you do. Or, if you want to improve your ability to squat on your heels or run with ease, you can keep a diary of the stretches you do and rate your ability to squat or run out of 10 (10 being the best) and you can also take photos and, or video clips on a regular basis. If you are writing your diary in a document on a computer, you can add the photos to the text.

The level of detail is also up to you. I recommend that you at least write down the stretches that you did and the number of reps, along with how you found them. If you would like to write more detail you can use a format like the one shown in Table 8.4.

Stretch	Reps	Notes (including range or motion, ease of movement, any modifications needed, etc.)	Quality of stretch /10
Child's pose	6	Stiff in my shoulders, could not go all the way down to having my head on the floor, feels challenging but like it's doing some good	5/10

Table 8.4 Example of an entry in a stretching diary

This allows you to write notes for each individual stretch, noting whatever you feel is relevant to you. The "Quality of stretch" section allows you to rate the stretch, and although this is very subjective, it serves to give you an idea of your improvement overall at a glance. So an 8/10 may mean that you feel comfortable, in control, and have a good range of motion in a stretch. A 2/10 may mean that it is hard, shaky, or you dislike doing it. If you want to be very diligent, you could take the scores at different dates and plot them into a graph to see your progress visually. I imagine that the maths fans among you will be keen on this!

Now that you have an idea of how flexible you are and how you can measure your flexibility going forward, you only need to read the pre-stretching instructions and you are ready to get started!!

9 How to Stretch

Pretty much everything you need to know about how to stretch with resistance is covered in this handy section, covering stretching effectively and safely as well as practical considerations.

Because resistance stretching is quite different from other stretching techniques, it is important that you have a thorough understanding of the method before you start. This is especially important if you are well-versed in another technique as the rules will not be the same.

I recommend that you take your time to read these points before you get started, but if you are in a hurry, do make sure that at the minimum you read the safety guidelines before you start. Please note that most of this advice is specific to resistance stretching and that it is important to read it all the way through before you start to stretch.

Warming Up

Many clients ask if they should warm up before stretching and the short answer is yes, it is best to do so. Stretching too intensely from cold may lead to unnecessary damage to the tissue, stiffness later on, and possibly injury, so warming the muscles up and getting the blood flowing for a few minutes can make a massive difference to the results you get from your stretching. I recommend that at the minimum you warm up by stretching gently at first and increasing the intensity as you go, following the body's cues of how open and far it wants to go. As the stretching always involves strength it will not take you too long to warm up, but do bear in mind that you

may have to warm up each area from scratch as you stretch it. Therefore, even if your body becomes warm from the effort of stretching your upper body, when you move to your lower body it is best to ease into it, warming the muscles and fascia up before you stretch them more deeply.

The pros of warming up before stretching include reduced risk of strain and injury from stretching muscles that are not prepared, you are more in the mood to stretch, and you do not have to combat any stiffness you may have from being still for too long. The cons are that it is easier to overstretch warm muscles and also if you are warmed up from cardio exercise you may find that any endorphin-fuelled enthusiasm may lead you to overdo it, so please bear this in mind!

You can use any one, or a combination, of these methods to get your body warmed up and ready for your stretching.

1. Use the warm-up stretches

Do the warm up stretches gently at first by using only a little resistance, and then gradually building up the tension as you feel your muscles becoming warmer, more ready, and more pliable. I recommend that you then progress to the more specific stretches when you feel warmed up and looser.

2. Warm up for stretching by stretching

Do any of the stretches with a gentle to medium level of resistance, giving your muscles time to get used to what you are doing and getting the blood circulating. As your body warms, you can increase the tension to stretch with more and more resistance.

While you are warming up you want to keep everything smooth, easy, and consistent and I suggest you avoid the stretches that you find very challenging.

3. Do 5 minutes of gentle exercise

This fits in particularly well if you are planning to do cardio, such as running, and want to stretch first. Doing your stretching 5 minutes into your workout means that you are warmed up enough and you will be able to experience the benefits of your stretching during your run/bike/exercise class/swim also. And stretching in a swimming pool (in the shallow end) is great fun because you can do a lot of movements without gravity getting in the way. If you are not doing any cardio, then 5 minutes of any movement that is safe and gets your whole body moving and warm, will work. Dancing is great too.

4. Warming up with warmth

Becoming physically warm by using a sauna, heating, or even living in a hot country, can also make us more ready to stretch. Popularized by hot yoga, stretching in a warm environment can make it easier to stretch as our tissues are already more supple and relaxed. Please be very careful not to overstretch if you do want to try this, make sure that you stay hydrated, and if you sweat make sure that you do not accidentally hurt yourself by slipping or losing your grip. I do not recommend stretching in a sauna because resistance stretching is more muscle-intensive and so it generates quite a lot of heat by itself. However, some people report good effects from having a 5 minute sauna before they stretch. This is an individual preference; personally I would rather warm up through exercise, as the body is in more of an active state then, which is more appropriate for such an involved technique. I do not recommend a heated environment if it makes you at all dizzy or "spaced-out", as you need to be able to concentrate to resistance stretch safely.

How Long Should I Warm-Up For?

The extent to which you need to warm up depends very much on your body in terms of how conditioned it is and how it reacts to physical exercise, as well as whether you "run hot" or "run cold" (the latter usually need to warm up for longer). If you know that you normally get stiff if you exercise without a warm-up then this will be especially true for your stretching. If you can run from cold without injury or stiffness then you may not need to warm up as much for your stretching, but please be aware that if the stretches are quite different to your usual movement routine, your body may not be as conditioned for them as you might expect, therefore, even if you are fit, you will still need to do a decent warm-up.

Generally I would say that if you are doing a longer, more intensive stretching session it would be good to spend at least 10 minutes warming up with any of the above methods. However, if you only want to do a 10-minute routine, you can warm up by doing the first few reps of each stretch more gently, and increasing the resistance as you warm up.

Engaging the Fascia

In order to affect our fascia we need it to be engaged throughout the movement, otherwise we will just be waving our limbs and torso back and forth without any effect. Fascia only becomes really actively involved in movement (although it is always holding and supporting us) when we create tension in our muscles.

The theory behind this is that fascia offers back-up strength to muscles, making us stronger in eccentric movements (in which muscles and fascia together are the "brakes") than in concentric strength movements (which muscles have to mainly make on their own). Therefore when we make an eccentric movement to stretch, the fascia is engaged and benefits from it, just like when we yawn, tense, and stretch first thing in the morning.

For even more benefit, when you are a little more experienced at resistance stretching, try visualizing that you are engaging the whole body while you tense and move as we are always working on the whole system, the whole body, as everything is connected. The more you work on the whole body with each movement, the greater and more widespread the changes will be.

How Hard Should I Resist?

Generating the correct level of tension in the muscles should allow us to move smoothly yet with some effort. It is enough to create a challenge to moving, but a level of challenge that is pleasurable to our bodies. Another way to describe it is as feeling like more of a joint effort than a fight. Often people who are new to resistance stretching think that tensing their muscles with 100% of their effort will yield the best results, but actually the best effect is achieved by creating a healthy and useful level of resistance. Becoming completely rigid in order to try to become more flexible and relaxed does not work. As a general rule we would say resist with 60–70% of your maximum ability.

Learning how much resistance is optimal is mainly done through practice and listening to your body, finding out what works through trial and error. If you are very sore and tired after stretching then you probably either resisted too much or did too much stretching. If you do not feel like you have stretched and are not moving more freely or feeling taller, then you have probably not resisted enough. It is important to note that if you are not quite as strong as you could be then you may ache as if you've had a workout afterwards, and that is completely natural.

The Correct Range of Motion

As previously mentioned, the ROM is shorter in resistance stretching. There are a couple of different possible signs that we have arrived at the end of our range. One sign is that you come to a point when you can no longer maintain the same level of tension, which decreases noticeably. Another sign is that you can maintain the tension but you feel like you have hit a brick wall and can go no further. If you start to feel discomfort or pain that is a kind of enforced end to the range of motion, as we do not stretch through pain.

When you reach the end of the ROM, do not go beyond this point, but continue to repeat the stretch and you will find that the range increases naturally. Remember, we are seeking sustainable increases in flexibility rather than trying to force our bodies to lengthen.

Timing, Duration, and Frequency of Stretching Sessions

Many clients who are new to stretching want to know when they should stretch, how long for, and how often. This is very specific to the individual, but here are some ideas for stretching plans, which you can experiment with:

- Daily morning stretching routine for 15–30 min
- Daily evening stretching routine for 15–30 min
- Stretching session every other day for 30–40 min
- 20-minute session 4 days a week and a 1-hour session 1 day a week
- 15–30 minutes after your normal workouts
- Stretching throughout the day whenever you can fit it in
- A combination of the above

I recommend that you do not jump into stretching all day every day unless you already have a highly conditioned body that is used to moving for long periods of time. Even so, resistance stretching is a strong form of stretching, so it is still advisable to build up slowly and find out what the optimum amount for your body is. Once you are more used to it you can stretch for long amounts of time (around 3 hours, for example) if you take it easy and do not push through pain or fatigue.

Stretching as a Warm-up for Sport

I find that stretching 5 minutes into an exercise session can be beneficial for people who are "naturally inflexible." It seems to improve the quality of their movements and make them feel easier and more fluid. This is especially the case for people who sit for most of the day, as suddenly expecting to be able to run, for example, with an open and balanced posture, after being folded up for hours, is asking a lot of the body. Most office workers who have exercised immediately after work will know that the body can feel stiff and resistant at first. Resistance stretching helps to alleviate the stiffness before putting all that force through our muscles.

However, there have been some studies showing that stretching before exercise can actually lead to increased risk of injury and decreased performance. For example, one study found that there was a decrease in power and performance in sprinters less than 30 minutes after static stretching. I believe this is because in static stretching, where you stay at the very end of your range of motion and attempt to push beyond it, you create slackness in your body by increasing the range of motion without also increasing strength. This impairs joint stability and the elastic recoil of your tissue impacting on biomechanics and performance. Obviously this is not useful when sprinting or performing other explosive exercises, where a higher degree of muscle tension is required in order to generate the power needed.

However, resistance stretching has a much shorter range of motion and actively strengthens muscles, and therefore I believe it is much less likely to cause inefficiency and instability. Although there have not yet been any studies on the effect of resistance stretching on power output and efficiency, many high-level athletes use resistance stretching to boost their performance. One such athlete is Dara Torres, an Olympic swimmer who discovered resistance stretching and then went on to win three silver medals at the age of 41. At one point whilst training she was getting stretched five times a day without losing power in her stroke (but I do not recommend that you try this unless you have a lot of experience of stretching and a very well conditioned body).

I recommend that if you are an athlete and would like to see how resistance stretching fits best into your training, try it for yourself at a few different times: a few hours before training, 40 minutes or more before you train, straight after training, and a few hours after training. Pay attention to how you feel, your times (and other measurements of performance), and your recovery. If you want to take it very seriously you can stretch at a specific time (in relation to your training) for a few days and keep a journal to monitor the benefits. It will depend on your sport, your schedule and your unique body, but when you find out what works for you, you will likely experience improvements in power, movement, recovery, and energy. Because many of the benefits to performance come from improved biomechanics and physical functioning, you do not need to do the stretches immediately before training. You can also stretch after your training session or at other points in the day as the effect of stretching regularly builds over days, weeks and months, rather than running out after 30 minutes.

For the rest of us who have more humble sporting aspirations, it is still a great idea to figure out when you get the best results from your stretching in terms of the time of day and how close to your exercise sessions you do it.

How to Stretch Safely

Although resistance stretching is very safe, there are some important points to note in order to avoid injury and get the best results.

Warm-up

As I mentioned before, by warming up you greatly reduce the risk of over-straining and being sore after stretching, as well as increase the ease and effectiveness of your stretching session.

It is strong stretching

Resistance stretching is also a form of strength training, so it is important to begin more gently at first, especially if you do not normally exercise very much, so that your body has a chance to become more conditioned. If you do it too intensely right away it is likely that you will be a bit achy afterwards, but this is not the same for everyone. If you are a bit sore, make sure that you drink enough water and keep moving through the day. A salt bath may help to relieve any muscle soreness.

Keep the tension on and stay within the healthy ROM

Another positive aspect of resistance stretching is that the tension that provides the resistance is protective, ensuring that the force is fairly evenly distributed throughout all of the tissues, avoiding excessive strain to any particular structures (as mentioned previously in Chapter 1) as well as stopping you from going beyond your natural range of motion. Therefore, it is important that you do maintain that tension throughout the stretch.

Often, because people find that the tension limits how far they can go in a movement, they relax their muscles enough to allow them to go further. However, the healthy range of motion in resistance stretching is specifically the distance that you can go whilst maintaining that tension (as long as there is no pain or discomfort). There is no benefit to doing these stretches without resistance and you can easily strain something by pushing beyond your natural limits.

Resist safely

Apart from remembering to resist, it is also important to remember not to resist too much. Although I mentioned this earlier in the chapter, I would like to reiterate that it is important to moderate your level of resistance. Many people think that tensing with all of their might gets the best results, but actually you need to resist much less at the beginning and gradually increase the intensity as you warm up. The most force you need to generate at any time is around 60–70% off your maximum resistance, or in other words, tense your muscles to around 60–70% of your strongest effort.

Stretch slowly

Because we are loading the muscles, using more force than in other techniques, and engaging all of the tissue types, we need to move more slowly whilst stretching. Similarly to the old adage of going at the speed of the slowest member of a group, we also need to do this whilst stretching our different tissues as some of them take longer to stretch healthily than others. Fascia in particular likes to stretch slowly, like, as Tom Myers says, a plastic bag that will tear when pulled quickly, but that can manage to stretch when pulled slowly.

Stretch smoothly with the correct amount of resistance

Very occasionally I have taught people who have initially stretched with harsh, jerky or excessively forceful movements. Sometimes they resist so much that they are shaking and the huge amount of force is so hard to move against that it makes the whole movement erratic. Through learning to use the correct level of resistance they now make smooth, even, graceful, and natural movements, which are so much more beneficial to the body.

Too much tension does not facilitate healthy change, but rather leads to soreness, restriction, and even less flexibility than before. We do not want the body to feel like it has to tense to protect itself, but to feel that it is safe, so that it allows itself to change and adapt rather than having to resist change to protect itself against injury.

Changing safely

Sometimes when the body has changed sufficiently that it can sustain a healthy change in alignment, one or several joints may "click" back into place. Although this is often very satisfying to people, and healthy when the body does it on its own steam, we do not try to make the body click intentionally. We risk causing injury if we try to get a click to happen by ourselves, because we may use too much force, strain ourselves, or create a change before the soft tissue is ready to support the body in that alignment. Trust that the body knows what it is right for it and do not "chase the click."

Stretch to your own ability

Although we have photos for you to follow, these are a guide only. Everyone's body is different, therefore how much strength you have and your ROM are unique to you. Practically this means that you may not be able to go as far as the model in the photo, or you may be able to go further. Use the guidelines for judging your end of ROM, not the photos, or even how far your friends can go!

If you have a little difficulty balancing for the standing stretches, many of them can be done while holding onto a chair. It is much better to do a stretch more gently while holding onto a chair than to risk falling over. I do not recommend taking any risks in order to stretch; you must always feel safe.

If you have any physical challenges then you may need to modify the stretches according to your needs. If you have difficulty doing so, I recommend erring on the side of caution and consulting a personal trainer or stretching trainer who may be able to help. Because the range of physical challenges varies, it is hard to make specific recommendations, but I would say listen to your body and maybe try shorter sessions at first to see how your body responds.'

How Can I Stretch If I Am in Pain?

If you have an existing pain in your body then please do check with your doctor or physiotherapist before starting to stretch. If you are fine to stretch but you find that the pain feels worse when you tense to create resistance, then I recommend trying these simple tips:

- Stay aware of the sore area and try to keep it relaxed while you stretch.

- Engage your abdominal muscles while you stretch and feel like the tension you need in the area you are stretching is coming from there, rather than the sore area.

- Use less tension so that it does not hurt to stretch (you may find that the soreness eases off naturally as you release your fascia and as your body warms up).

- Keep breathing all throughout the movement and, as I said before, do not stretch with a no-pain, no-gain attitude.

- If you have any tense and inflamed muscles it is best not to stretch them directly, but stretch around them and actively avoid tensing them even when stretching other areas.

If in doubt, do not stretch, but check with a professional or stretching trainer first.

After Your First Few Resistance Stretching Sessions

Resistance stretching always involves strength, so it is completely normal to feel slightly (or even very) achy after your first few sessions or an intense session, as if you have worked out. This is a great sign that you have been strengthening areas that could be stronger and the only way through is to keep going. Do not give up just because of some aching muscles; keep moving, drink enough water, and try a sea salt bath to relieve the muscle ache. As a side note, please note that muscle ache is one thing, but if you experience any sharp or worrying pains then stop stretching until you have consulted a doctor.

You will not have muscle ache after all of your sessions and in the future it may never ever happen, but when you start to use your body in a new way it is common for it to complain a little. If you are not achy, that is fine too. It may mean that your body is naturally resilient and likes stretching, or that you have already conditioned your body enough through exercise and movement.

It is highly likely that your friends will notice improvements in your movement, posture, looks, and even height, and will ask you what you have been doing. If you let them in on your secret you could start stretching with them perhaps. Please do refer them to this book or our website so they can learn how to stretch powerfully and safely and do not try to teach people yourself unless you have passed one of our Moving Stretch® training qualifications.

Practical Considerations

What you will need

It is beneficial to have a yoga mat, a yoga strap, and some comfy clothes; in addition, some of the stretches require a doorway, a chair, or a desk. However, if you are lacking any of these things, you can substitute others that you have at hand. For example, sometimes a staircase is a good substitute for a desk and a wall can be a substitute for the doorway.

If you do not have a yoga mat, you can do the lying-down stretches on your bed or on the floor on the carpet or a towel (be careful of slipping on smooth flooring), and do the standing stretches on the floor. If you need extra protection for your knees you can use a towel. If you do not have a yoga strap, then a pair of non-stretchy trousers will do the job. Simply use the bit where the legs join, as a substitute for the mid-point of a yoga strap and grasp the ankles together with your hands. If you do not have trousers, then a towel or belt will do instead.

You may also want a notebook and pen if you decide to keep a stretching diary.

Where you can stretch

Everywhere. I stretch on public transport, at bus stops, whilst doing the washing up. The only limitations are probably on roads, whilst driving a car, or operating heavy machinery. (I have had a quick stretch on my bicycle but I do not recommend it!) If you are at work why not try the seated stretches in the specific office-based routine, or if you need somewhere more private you can do a couple of the standing poses somewhere like a bathroom cubicle, but just be careful about loud sighs of relief!

You may feel foolish, but if you wait to be somewhere where it is socially acceptable to stretch, you will be waiting for most of your day unless you happen to be at home, in the gym, or in a park. Also, you never know who you may inspire to move more, just by seeing you do a quick stretch at the desk or the bus stop.

Now, if you are ready, it is time to get our stretch on!

10   The Moving Stretches

I have organized these stretches into five main categories for ease of use:

- whole-body and warm-up stretches
- stretches for the front of the body
- stretches for the back of the body
- stretches for the outside of the body
- stretches for the inside of the legs

These stretches are laid out according to the area of the body they focus on, rather than specific muscles or muscle groups. There are some exceptions to this, but the reason it is set out this way is that we are focusing on working with the fascia, and focusing on specific muscles would not help, and might even hinder, your stretching. In addition, a system this simple is easy for everyone to use; you do not need to know all of the names of the muscles or be an expert on anatomy to find a stretch and use it. For the sake of simplicity, the names of the stretches are also very straightforward (although it might have been more fun to give them names like "Flabbergasted Fox Flying" I realized that I and others would have to actually remember them, and as there are 95 stretches that might be a bit of a challenge), with most of names describing the movement aspect of the stretch or the area being stretched.

Occasionally I list the main muscle(s) associated with a stretch, but this does not mean that the effect of the stretch is limited to that exact area. The fascia connects the entire body and when stretching it is not unusual to feel benefits as far away as the face when stretching the legs, for example.

It is more common for a stretch on the front of the thighs to affect the front of the body more than the back, but due to the interconnected nature of the body, there can be knock-on benefits throughout the body, even where least expected. For example, one of my clients experiences a release in the pressure of her sinuses each time she stretches her quads, so it is great to be open to trying different stretches and observe what works for you.

Let us also briefly recap some of the key points on how to stretch before you start:

1. You need to resist in order to benefit from each stretch. Resist by creating tension in your muscles, which will automatically generate tension in your fascia. This allows you to work on the fascia while you make each movement. Do not drop the resistance at any point and make sure you have created the tension before you move at all.

2. Resisting the movement may feel a bit counterintuitive at first. Usually resistance is created by the part being stretched trying to go in the opposite direction or to resist the movement in general.

3. Do not resist to your maximum strength (going as stiff as a plank) as you will tire out very quickly, probably feel sore afterwards, and possibly also injure yourself. I recommend that you try tensing your muscles at around 60–70% of their maximum ability. You can increase or decrease this as needed, but as a general rule you should be able to move smoothly, without pain, and without a grimace on your face, but not so easily that you can forget what you are doing.

4. Avoid over-stretching by listening to the body. If you cannot continue along that line of movement with the same amount of resistance then you have come to the end of that stretch. Remember that the range of motion (ROM) during a Moving Stretch is smaller than in other stretches, such as static stretches, due to the effect of the resistance on the structure of the body. So rather than pushing beyond your healthy range, simply relax and start again.

5. Do not push through pain. This is not a no-pain, no-gain scenario. You want to work with your body to find out what it needs, so try working around your issue to find relief instead of trying to force some kind of release.

6. Do not focus on the end of the ROM. Moving Stretch is all about *moving* (as well as resistance), so although it can be hard to let go of our results-oriented desire to go as far as possible, that is not where our stretch actually happens. The stretch happens while you are moving in a healthy ROM and that is where the fascia is reconditioned also.

7. All of these stretches are Moving Stretches, which means they always involve movement. The stretch actually happens during the movement and we do not wait at the end of the ROM, but return to the starting position.

8. We want to make smooth, steady movements and avoid jerking and fast or sudden movements.

Rather than trying to remember to tense each individual muscle, try thinking about tensing one or two aspects of the body, such as the front of the thigh and the abdomen. I give specific instructions about where to create tension for each stretch and you will get the most benefit from tensing those areas at the same time, unless stated otherwise.

If you find it hard to think about tensing several areas at once, then you can try thinking about making the movement hard for yourself. For example, if you are going to lean forward, then by tensing everything that will make that movement difficult, you will be tensing the muscles on the back of your body.

Remember that if you are using these stretches to warm up, then you have to ease yourself into it. When you start, make the movements more gently, with shorter distances and with less resistance. As you warm up you can increase the amount of resistance you are using, and how far you are moving.

The number of repetitions is only a rough guide; if you are tired straight away then starting with 3 is fine and if you are über-fit you may be able to do 20 or more right away. Listen to your body and try not to get carried away, especially for your first few sessions, as you may be sore later. It is a good idea to do the recommended amount of reps and change to another stretch or two before coming back and doing another set.

You can, of course, move through any and all of these stretches, but I suggest that you create a balanced stretching session by following these general guidelines:

- Ease into your session with a few whole-body, warm-up stretches.

- Alternate between stretches for the back and front, outside and inside, top and bottom of your body.

- Do at least one stretch per session that you find difficult (and feel like avoiding).

- Start with gentle resistance and increase the intensity as you warm up.

- Always move with resistance in your muscles and fascia by creating tension and do not let that tension go, especially not in order to be able to go further in a stretch.

- Have a back-up routine (which you can adapt as needed from week to week, or month to month) that takes care of all your most pressing needs, for days when you are too tired to think about what to do.

- Enjoy yourself. Be experimental, be playful, and try letting your instinct pick which stretch you do next. It can be a wonderful experience and you will not feel like you are stretching because you "should," but rather because you "can."

- It is not always the most obviously tight or sore area that needs to be stretched, as often this is just a symptom of an issue somewhere else. Of course, if you have a physical issue that is causing you pain or not resolving itself it is important to see a professional such as a doctor or physiotherapist. However, if you are trying to troubleshoot an issue on your own I recommend that you gently and consistently work through the stretches in the areas surrounding your issue, rather than just that specific area, and prioritize the stretches that you find difficult because the ROM is limited, even if you do not feel any soreness there. For example, if you have very tight hips and pain in your glutes, try stretching the outside, inside, and front of your hips instead of focusing on the back of your hips where the pain is.

- If you want to make your own personalized routine and need some inspiration, have a look at the stretching routines featured later in this book for ideas.

And now for the stretches. Take your time with them, and enjoy!

General Warm-Up Stretches

These stretches are amazing for waking up in the morning, warming up for stretching or exercise, or just to wind down from a busy day. They get the body moving as a whole, increasing blood and lymph circulation, warming the muscles up, and also get you in the mood for stretching.

Aim to be gentle and relaxed, while keeping the body engaged. Do not tense your muscles 100%, but ease into the movements; the focus is to warm up rather than to stretch strongly. You can increase the amount of tension in your muscles as you get more warmed up.

Although you do not need to do all of them, I recommend that you do them roughly in the order given as the more general, whole-body stretches are at the beginning and then the ones toward the end are targeted to more specific areas. Because they do involve a larger area than some of the more specific stretches that we cover later on, it is important to create tension in a lot of muscles at once.

> **Note**: If you start your session with a few warm up stretches, it can be a great idea to do a couple of the same warm-up stretches again at the end of your session. Why? Because there are few things that reflect your changes back to you as well as a specific movement such as a stretch. See if it is easier to do these stretches at the end of your stretching session, and also notice whether your posture has changed and how you feel different. You may notice a difference in range of motion, ease of movement, fluidity, balance or co-ordination for example.

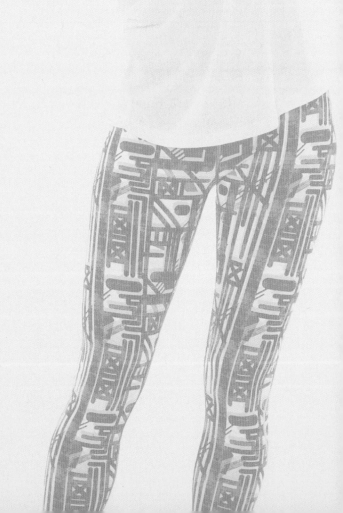

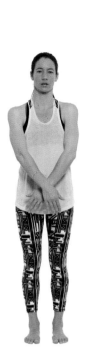
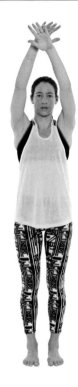
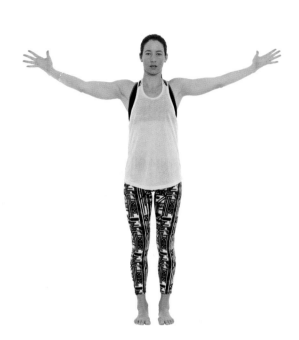

Main area and muscles stretched
Stretches the chest and upper body.

Technique
Stand with your feet shoulder-width apart and cross your hands over in front of your hips. Tensing your abdomen, chest, and the front of your shoulders, lift your arms up and out in front of you, up the midline of the body and over your head. At the very top, start to separate your hands and continue to tense your chest and shoulders as you draw a wide circle out and down with your fingertips. At the end of the circle, come back to the starting position.

Technique tips
Lead with a different finger for each repetition; i.e., the forefinger pushing out the most, then next time the middle finger, etc. When you come to your thumb have a very open hand.

This is a great warm-up stretch that opens your chest and shoulders and gets the blood flowing right away. Think about opening up and stretching out in all directions with your arms.

Suggested number of reps in one set
6; one with the whole hand, and then one with each different finger leading.

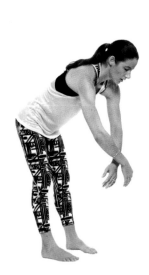
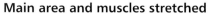
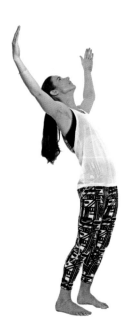

Main area and muscles stretched
On the way back; your abdomen, chest, the front of your shoulders and the front of your hips.

On the way forward; your back and the back of your hips.

Technique
Stand with your hips shoulder-width and a half apart. Tense the front of your hips, abdomen, and chest and simultaneously pull your arms up, out (at 45° from your midline) and back, and push your hips forward, stretching your chest, abdomen, and front of your hips.

Now tense the muscles of your back and the back of your shoulders and hips as you bring your arms down and in front of you and push your middle and lower back out behind you, leaning forward slightly, and curling your body inward. One repetition includes moving backward and forward once.

As you warm up, expand the stretch to include your hamstrings by tensing the backs of your legs and leaning forward from your hips as shown.

Technique tips
The purpose of this stretch is to stretch the whole front of your body by pushing your hips forward and arching your body backward, and a lot of the back of your body by bending forward and reaching forward with your arms. Think of curling and uncurling yourself. This stretch requires a bit of strength, which is a bonus in terms of warming you up.

Suggested number of reps in one set
7–10.

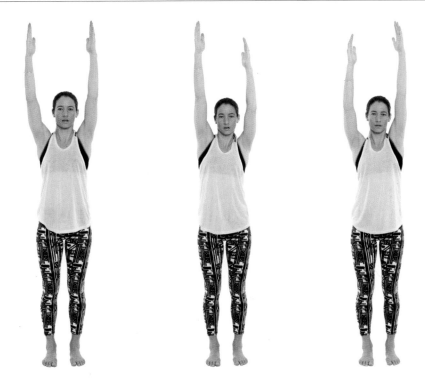

Main area and muscles stretched
Stretches your back and around your ribs.

Technique
Stand with your feet a little closer than shoulder-width apart. Raise your hands out to the sides and up and, as you do so, imagine a line between your hands passing up through your body. As the line passes up through your muscles, tense each muscle that it passes through.

With your arms parallel, tense the sides of your torso and the muscles around your ribs and back as you pull one arm higher than the other. Hold for a moment then repeat on the other side.

Technique tips
Although this is a stretch with only a small movement, it packs a punch.

By reaching up on one side against tension, you can stretch a lot of the fascia and deeper muscles in your torso, even around your spine and ribs. Think about reaching up, not sideways.

Suggested number of reps in one set
5–7 on each side.

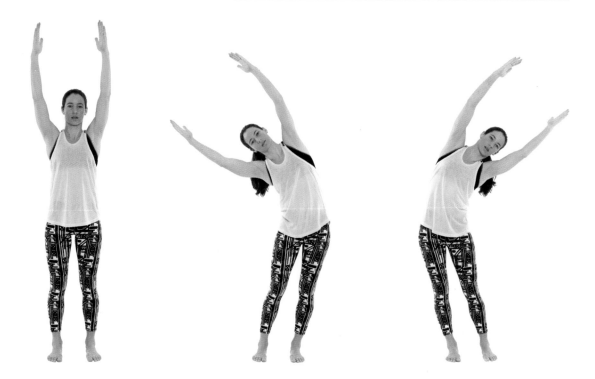

Main area and muscles stretched
Your side and the outside of your hip (on the same side).

Technique
Stand with your feet a little closer than shoulder-width apart. Raise your hands out to the sides and up and, as you do so, imagine a line between your hands passing up through your body. As the line passes up through your muscles, tense each muscle that it passes through.

Reach up to the sky with parallel arms, tense your sides and abdomen and reach to one side as you push your opposite hip out in the other direction, curving yourself like a bow.

Remember to keep the muscles of your torso engaged all the time. Return to the center and then push to the other side.

Technique tips
You will be stretching one side of your torso at a time, all the way down to your hip and even down the outside of your leg.

You are thinking about tensing all of those areas as you lean in the opposite direction. When you lean you are curving yourself sideways like a bow. Be careful if you have any back issues and if you find this stretch hard it is fine to place one hand on your hip, of the side you are moving towards, to support you.

Suggested number of reps in one set
5 on each side.

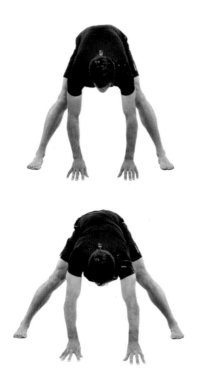

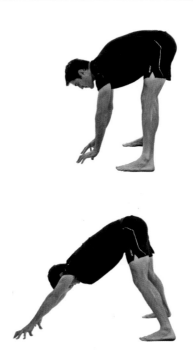

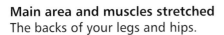

Main area and muscles stretched
The backs of your legs and hips.

Technique
Stand with your legs wide apart and fold yourself in half as you lower your hands to the floor, keeping your abdominal muscles engaged on the way down to support your back.

Continuously tense the backs of your legs, as you walk your hands forward as far as you can comfortably and then back towards you and then between your legs as far as you can without falling on your bottom. Walking your hands forward and backward once is one rep.

Technique tips
This exercise stretches the backs of your legs, and by walking forward and backward with your hands and tensing your hamstrings you can recondition old, tight, or stuck fascia in the backs of your legs.

The key is to keep the tension on in the backs of your legs and to only go as far as you can comfortably go.

Suggested number of reps in one set
6–9.

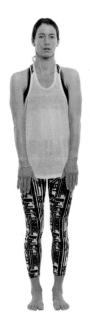 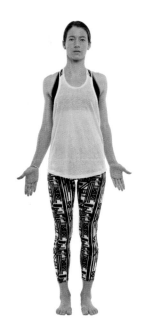 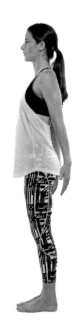

Main area and muscles stretched
Stretches the chest and the upper back

Technique
In this stretch the arms rotate around you, with your palms always facing the body. Start with your arms straight down and in front of the body, palms facing your thighs. Tensing your chest and shoulders, move your arms out and around behind you to stretch your chest. Then tensing your back and especially the muscles between your shoulder blades, move your arms back around to the front again, stretching your upper back. Keep your hands close to your body. Moving your arms backward and then forward counts as one rep.

Technique tips
This stretch is unusual in that you stretch in both directions, so it is really two stretches rolled into one. Because of this you have to remember to keep the resistance on in the correct area in order for the stretch to work.

Suggested number of reps in one set
7–10.

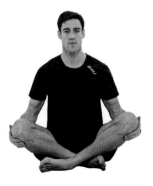 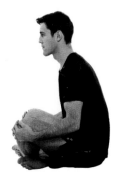

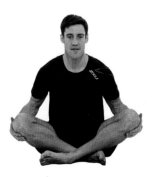 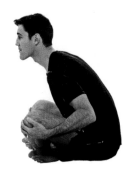

Main area and muscles stretched
Stretches the abductors.

Technique
Sit with your legs crossed and hands under your knees. Push your knees down into your hands continuously as you lean forward to stretch. Make sure your feet are not too far back toward your bottom but roughly under your knees; play with the distance so that you feel a stretch.

Technique tips
If you are naturally flexible make sure your feet are far enough forward in order to get a stretch in your abductors. If you are very stiff then do not worry if your knees are very high. You can also move your feet further from your body if that is easier, and do not push too hard or lean forward further than is comfortable.

Suggested number of reps in one set
7–10.

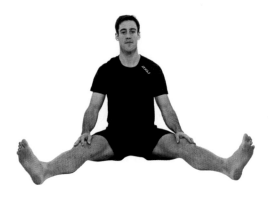

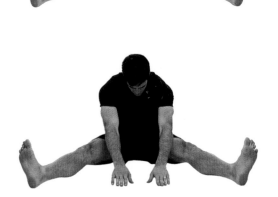

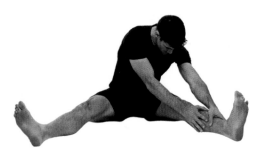

Main area and muscles stretched
The backs and insides of your thighs, groin and lower back.

Technique
Sit with your legs as wide apart as is comfortable for you. Have your toes pointing up to the sky throughout the whole stretch.

Pull your feet down into the ground continuously as you reach for one foot (it's OK to hold your knee or calf if you can't reach your foot) and hold for a second before returning to the middle and reaching for the other foot, hold for a second, and then reach straight forward in front of you.

Technique tips
Remember to keep the tension on by pulling your feet into the floor. You do not need to go very far, necessarily, in order to get a good stretch so do not worry about hunching your back over in order to go further. Focus on rocking your hips in the direction that you are leaning, rather than making up for a smaller range of motion by reaching out with your arms as that will not help and may make your back tight.

This stretch is a variation on an old classic, the only difference being that it is a Moving Stretch so you need to resist continuously and remember that most of the stretch happens while you are moving, so move slowly and you do not need to stay at the end of the range of motion for longer than one second.

Think about tensing the muscles on the inside as well as the back of the legs and keeping your back long.

The key is to keep the tension going in the backs of your legs and to only go as far as you can comfortably go.

Suggested number of reps in one set
7–9 in each direction.

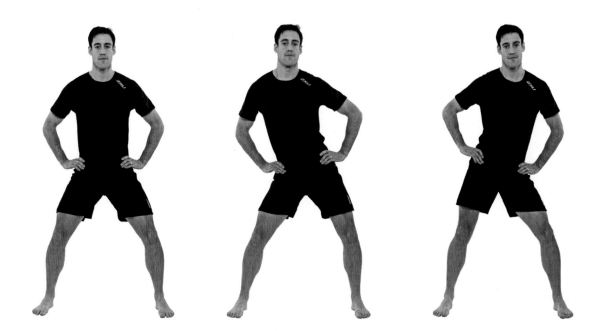

Main area and muscles stretched
Stretches the adductors.

Technique
Squat with your feet shoulder-width and a half apart and your bottom tucked underneath you. Tense the muscles of your hips (and especially the side in the direction you are moving) as you push your hips out to one side and slightly up in an arc. Then tense the other outer side of your thighs and push your hips toward that side in the same way, so that you are slowly rocking your hips from side to side.

Keep your bottom tucked under throughout the stretch.

Technique tips
Imagine the movement pattern you would make if you were rocking a baby from side to side in your arms. You want to make that movement but with your hips. Think about tensing the muscles on the inside as well as the back of the legs and keeping your back long. This stretch is great for opening and warming up the hips.

Suggested number of reps in one set
7–9 in each direction.

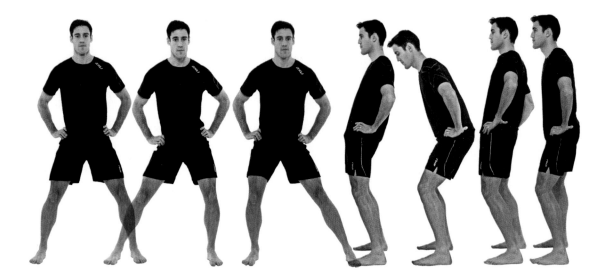

Main area and muscles stretched
Stretches the hips.

Technique
Stand with your feet hip-width apart. You are going to move your hips in eight directions out from the center point in the middle of your body, as if you were following the points of a compass. Before you move your hips, tense the muscles on the side of the body in the direction you are going. For example, before you push your hips straight out to the left, continuously tense the muscles on the outside of the left hip, as well as all of the muscles around your hips, upper thighs, back, and lower abdomen.

These are the directions you will stretch: to the left side, to the right side, forward, backward (do not stick your bottom out, but keep your hips tucked under and push your tailbone backward), diagonally forward and left, diagonally backward and right and then the reverse; diagonally forward and right, diagonally backward and left.

Technique tips
It can be hard to keep your tailbone tucked under if you are not used to it. You can think of it as trying to keep the small of your back as straight as possible. Keeping your hands on your hips to guide you so that you can feel what your hips are doing or watching yourself in a mirror may be a good idea.

This stretch is one of the most challenging for people co-ordination-wise, not least because many people in the West cannot really move their hips, let alone in multiple directions. Which is a great reason not to avoid this stretch.

Suggested number of reps in one set
5 in each direction in total.

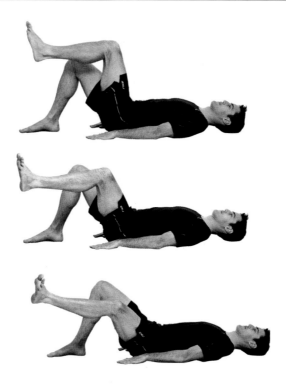

Main area and muscles stretched
Stretches the abductors.

Technique
Lie on your back and lift your leg up into the air, so that your knee is above your hip, with your knee bent at 90°. Tense all of the muscles in and around your hips as you slowly rotate your knee to the outside and down to the midline of your body, and back up again in a circle.

Technique tips
Try to keep your hips flat on the floor and keep your core engaged so that you don't wobble from side to side. Keeping your other knee bent should help to keep the small of your back flat on the ground, but it is a good idea to press it gently into the ground as you do this stretch also.

Suggested number of reps in one set
7–10 on each side.

Front of the Body

These stretches are for the front of the neck, chest, torso and legs and help to open up the chest and hips. People generally tend to stretch the back of the body more than the front, as tension in the back is generally more obvious. However, when you start working through these stretches you may find that the front of your body is more tense than you'd expect.

Generally speaking, stretches for the front of the body need a little more of a warm up than those for the back of the body, so start with a little less tension in the muscles and build up to a normal amount. You may want to do the stretches a little more slowly as well initially, giving your body time to get into the swing of things. Stretching the front of your body can make you feel more open and balanced.

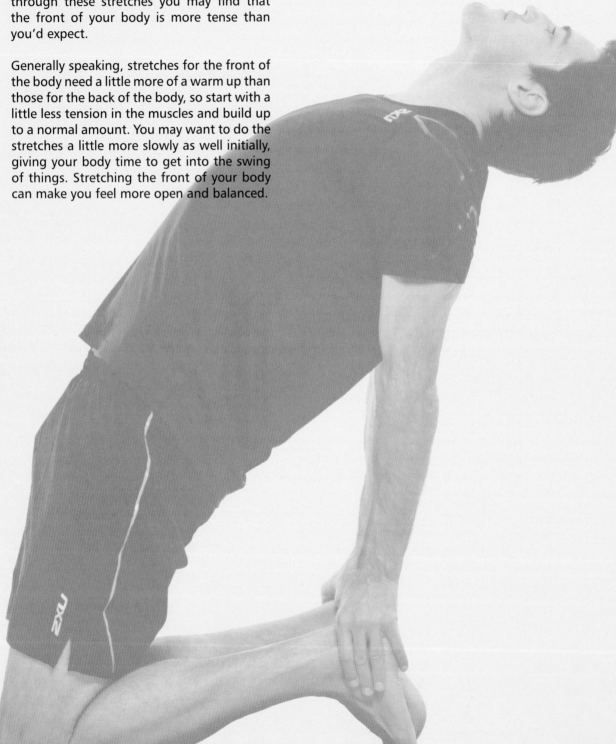

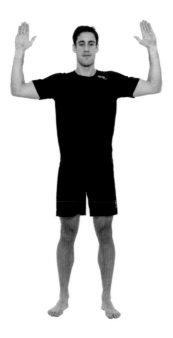
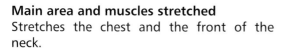
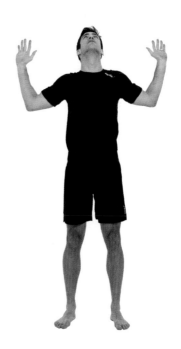

Main area and muscles stretched
Stretches the chest and the front of the neck.

Technique
Let your chin drop down to your chest and raise your arms, bent, to your sides and slightly in front of you. Tense the muscles of your chest, the front of your neck and front of your shoulders as you smoothly raise your head and pull your arms back against that resistance as far as it is comfortable to go. Lifting your head and arms back and then easily returning to the start position counts as one rep.

Technique tips
Keep the tension in the front of your neck only, rather than the back of your neck.

Suggested number of reps in one set
5–7.

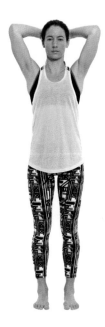
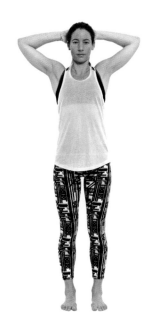

Main area and muscles stretched
Stretches the chest and shoulders.

Technique
With your hands clasped behind your head and your elbows forward and close to one another, tense your chest continuously and move your elbows back. Moving both elbows back once and returning easily to the beginning position is one rep.

Technique tips
Do not pull on your head with your hands or you may make your neck tense. Make the movement nice and smooth. You do not need to look up as you stretch, but keep your head level.

Suggested number of reps in one set
7–10.

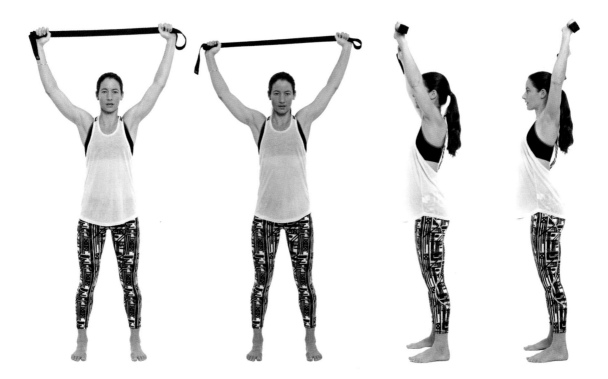

Main area and muscles stretched
Stretches the chest and shoulders.

Technique
Grip a yoga strap, belt, or towel above your head firmly in both hands. Your arms should form a "V" so try to make sure you are holding the strap in the correct position.

With your hands pulling continuously apart from each other to create tension, move your hands back behind you, keeping your elbows straight. When you have gone as far back as you can comfortably reach, return easily to the starting position to complete one rep.

Technique tips
If you get tired from having your arms above your head for so long it is fine to take a break mid-set. Also, if you are very flexible, only move your arms back as far as your shoulders stay in the same position in the joint—we do not want any contortionism in this stretch!

Suggested number of reps in one set
7–9.

4. CHEST STRETCH AT DESK

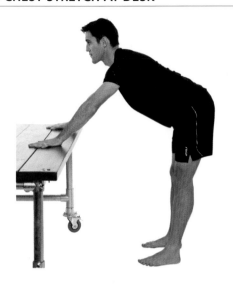 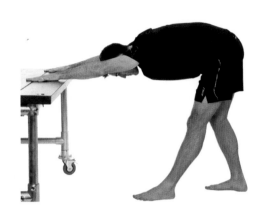

Main area and muscles stretched
Stretches the chest and the front of the shoulders as well as the upper back.

Technique
With your arms wide, place your hands on a desk and pull them down and inward, without moving them. Slowly lower yourself against that tension until your torso is parallel (or closer to parallel) to the ground. Return easily to the start and repeat.

Technique tips
Do not lean forward on your hands while you do this, as you would in a press-up, but keep the weight in your legs. Also try to keep your back flat and your shoulders down away from your ears.

Suggested number of reps in one set
7–9.

5. CHEST STRETCH ON CHAIR

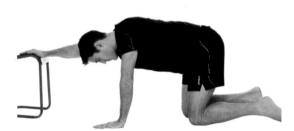 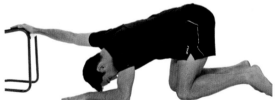

Main area and muscles stretched
Stretches the chest and inner arm.

Technique
Kneel with a chair in front of you and out to the side, one hand diagonally out, palm-down on the seat, pressing down continuously. Smoothly lean down to the floor to stretch your chest, by sitting back and bending your other arm.

Technique tips
If stretching with your arm straight hurts your elbow at all, just bend it slightly, and keep it bent like that throughout the stretch.

Suggested number of reps in one set
7–10 on each side.

6. PULLING ARM DOWN INTO FLOOR AND OPENING CHEST

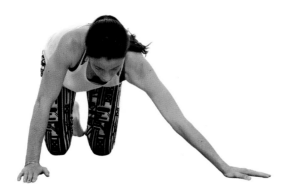 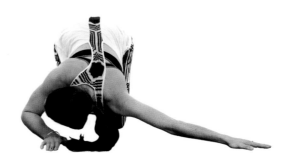

Main area and muscles stretched
Stretches the chest and inner arm.

Technique
On your hands and knees, put one arm straight out to the side, fingers pointing away from you. Pull it continuously down into the floor as you lower your upper body and twist your torso, looking away from your straight arm. Never stop pulling into the ground with the straight arm.

Technique tips
You can change the position of the arm out to the side, by moving your hand a few inches forward each time. Bear in mind that in order to stretch effectively in this instance, you always need to sit back away from your outstretched arm, wherever it is. This changes the area being stretched, giving you a more well-rounded stretch.

Suggested number of reps in one set
7–10 on each side.

7. PULLING BOTH ARMS DOWN INTO THE FLOOR

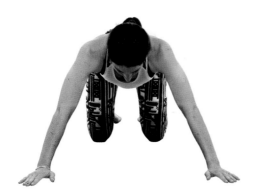 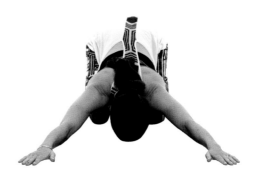

Main area and muscles stretched
Stretches the chest and inner arms.

Technique
On your hands and knees, put your arms straight out in front of you in a "V" shape, fingers pointing away from you. Pull your hands continuously down into the floor and back toward your body as you lower your upper body, stretching your chest and inner arms.

Technique tips
Make sure that you do not move down into a push-up, but sit backwards keeping your body weight off your arms as you pull them into the ground to engage your chest. This stretch also benefits the upper back, so don't worry if you feel the stretch there also.

Suggested number of reps in one set
7–10.

8. KNEELING PUSH-UP CHEST STRETCH

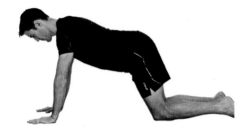 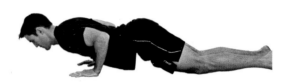

Main area and muscles stretched
Stretches the chest.

Technique
Get into a kneeling push-up with your hands wider than they usually would be. Create tension in your chest then let your chest fall toward the floor in slow motion, to stretch. Come up easily and quickly and repeat the stretch. One way to make it a little easier is to imagine "pulling" the floor toward you on your way down.

Technique tips
Visualize your shoulders becoming broader and your chest more open as you lower yourself down. If it is too hard to do 7–10 reps just start with 3–5 and build up.

Suggested number of reps in one set
7–9.

9. DOORWAY OPENING STRETCH

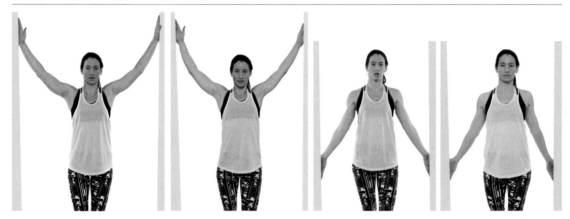

Main area and muscles stretched
Stretches the chest and inner arms.

Technique
Stand a little behind a doorway looking through it and raise your arms upward into a "V." Put your hands on the doorframe and push into it with a moderate pressure to create tension in your chest. Take one step forward through the doorway, maintaining the tension in your chest and shoulders and push through the doorway chest-first. Return easily and repeat.

Technique tips
You can also do this exercise with your arms in a downward "V" to stretch a different part of your chest.

Do not lean down and forward, but keep your head up and push your chest forward in a line parallel with the floor. Also only take one step, as if you take multiple steps it will break up the movement too much and you will not stretch your chest. Do not worry if your hands need to slide slightly on the doorframe to accommodate the movement, it is better that this happens than having to bend your elbows to move forward. As long as you keep your arms in a "V" all is well.

Suggested number of reps in one set
7–9.

10. PALMS ON FLOOR FOREARM STRETCH

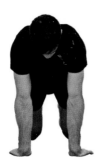 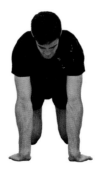

Main area and muscles stretched
Stretches the forearms and hands.

Technique
Get on to your hands and knees and turn your hands around so that your fingers are pointing back toward you with your thumbs out. Push your fingers down into the ground as you sit back slowly, stretching your hands and forearms, keeping your elbows as straight as you can comfortably hold them.

Technique tips
If you want to make this stretch less intense put your hands closer to your body and if you want to make it stronger move your palms further forward, away from your body. Do not make jerky or sudden movements or push through any pain.

Suggested number of reps in one set
5–7.

11. WRIST STRETCH AT DESK

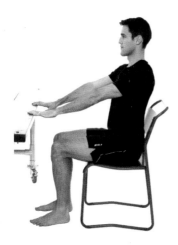 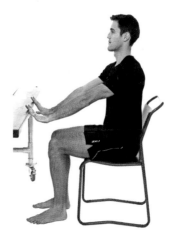

Main area and muscles stretched
Stretches your wrists and palms.

Technique
Rest your fingers on the edge of a desk and have your fingers and hands push down and into the desk. Lean forward with your body to push the heel of your palm forward and down, stretching your wrists and palms.

Technique tips
Only push as hard with your fingers as you can without causing discomfort and always keep your elbows straight.

Suggested number of reps in one set
7–10.

12. PULLING FINGERS DOWN STRETCH

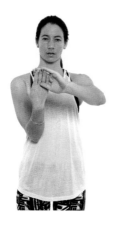
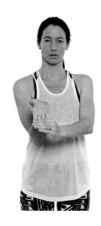

Main area and muscles stretched
Stretches the fingers, palms, and forearms.

Technique
Stand with your inner forearm and your palm facing toward you and your other hand resting across your fingers. As your fingers and palm pull toward you, your other hand pulls them smoothly away from you and down as far as they can go comfortably. Return easily to the starting position to complete one rep.

Technique tips
The key to this stretch is to make the movement very smooth.

Suggested number of reps in one set
5–7 on each hand.

13. PRAYER HANDS

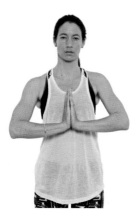
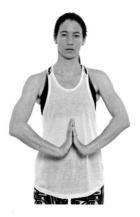

Main area and muscles stretched
Stretches the fingers, palms, and forearms.

Technique
Touching your palms together in front of your chest, push your fingers and thumbs together. Maintain that pressure as you evenly lower your hands, separating the heels of your palms to stretch your hands and fingers. Always keep the fingertips touching and the tension on and only go as far down as you are still getting a stretch. Return easily to the start position and repeat.

Technique tips
To alter the stretch keep pushing your fingers and palms together but do not lower your hands, as you move them so that your fingertips point first to one side and then the other, keeping the heels of your palms still and touching all the time.

Suggested number of reps in one set
7–10.

14. CLASPED-HANDS STRETCH

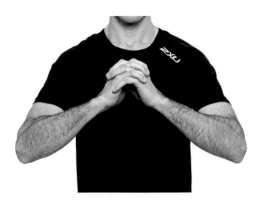 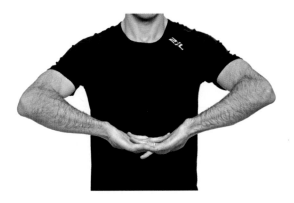

Main area and muscles stretched
Stretches your palms and fingers.

Technique
Clasp your hands with your palms touching. Squeeze your fingers together and spread and lower your palms smoothly and slowly as far as you can comfortably. Return easily to the starting position to complete one rep.

Technique tips
The aim is not to crack your knuckles, but if they do so naturally that is fine. Do not worry if you cannot go very low, just focus on maintaining the tension in the range that you can do. Be careful not to go too far, but only as far as you can keep the tension on.

Suggested number of reps in one set
7–10.

15. CLAW STRETCH

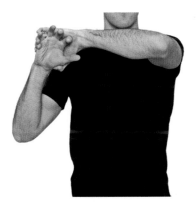 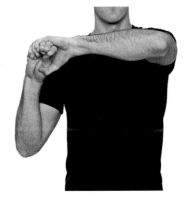

Main area and muscles stretched
Stretches your whole hand.

Technique
Make your hand into a claw-shape and tense all of the muscles in your hand and fingers. Squeeze your "claw" hand with your other hand and then release.

Technique tips
Similarly to some of the other hand stretches you may notice an increase in dexterity after stretching.

Suggested number of reps in one set
7–10 on each hand.

16. QUAD STRETCH ON KNEES

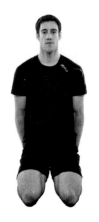 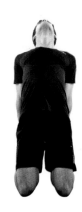 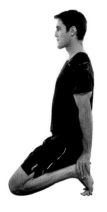 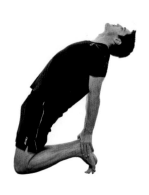

Main area and muscles stretched
Stretches the chest, abdomen, quads and hip flexors.

Technique
Kneel with your hands on your heels and sit on your heels with your shoulders pulled forward. Tense the front of your hips, your abdomen and chest as you sit up, pushing your hips forward and your shoulders back, always keeping your hands on your heels.

Technique tips
In order to stretch a larger area, you can also tense the front of your throat and move your elbows and head back when you push your hips forward, as far as you can comfortably go.

Suggested number of reps in one set
7–10.

17. HIP FLEXORS AT CHAIR

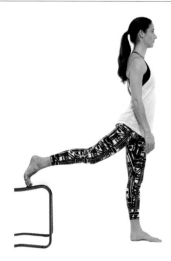 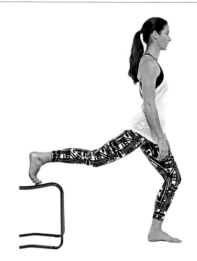

Main area and muscles stretched
Stretches the hip flexors.

Technique
Stand with a chair or step behind you and put your foot up on it. Keeping your back knee as straight as you comfortably can, pull your foot down into the chair to tense your muscles while you smoothly bend your standing leg to stretch. Come back up easily.

Technique tips
Try to keep your body upright as you complete the stretch.

Suggested number of reps in one set
7–10 on each side.

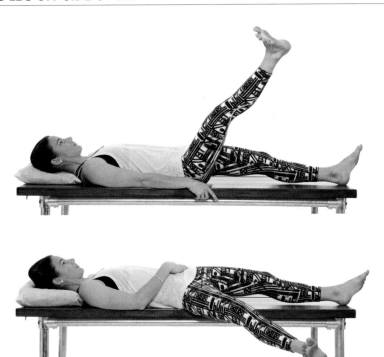

Main area and muscles stretched
Stretches the hip flexors.

Technique
Lie close to the side of a bed, sofa or solid table, with the leg closest to the side straight, slightly out to the side and up in the air. Hold onto something stable or put the arm furthest from the edge out to the side to counterbalance you to stop you rolling off.

Tensing the hip of your straight leg and your abdominal muscles, lower the leg slowly diagonally down and out, even passing down to below the level you are lying on if it is comfortable to do so.

Remember to always keep the tension on throughout the movement and also let yourself return to the starting position very easily, you can bend your leg if you prefer.

Technique tips
If your hip joint "clunks" when you lower your leg, try altering the angle that you are moving the leg down through, or the rotation of your leg, by pointing your toes outward more.

Suggested number of reps in one set
7–10 on each side.

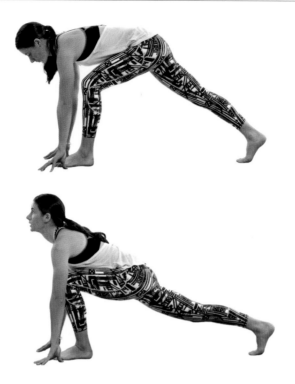

Main area and muscles stretched
Stretches the hip flexors.

Technique
Crouch as if you were getting into the starting position for a race, with both hands on the floor and then push your back leg even further out behind you so that your legs are quite far apart. Push your bottom up into the air and tense the front of your hips as you lower your hips down and lift your head as far as you can comfortably manage, bending your front knee even more.

Return easily to the start and repeat.

Technique tips
To generate even more resistance you can pull your back leg down into the ground and then move against that force. If this stretch is too difficult then you can kneel on one knee, pulling that knee forward as you lean forward, bending your front knee even more.

Suggested number of reps in one set
5–7 on each side.

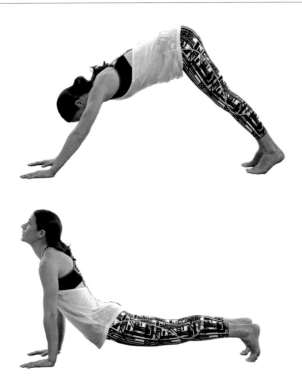

Main area and muscles stretched
Stretches the hip flexors and lower abdomen.

Technique
Get into a full push-up position, and push your hips high up into the air. Tensing the front of your hips and abdomen, lower your hips toward the ground against that continuous tension. Return to the starting position as easily as possible.

Technique tips
If this is too hard then you can do it in a kneeling push-up position, in which case you should let your feet point up into the air, placing padding under your knees if you need to.

Suggested number of reps in one set
Reps: 5–7.

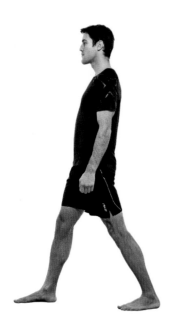
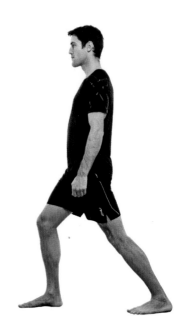

Main area and muscles stretched
Stretches the hip flexors.

Technique
Stand with one foot in front of the other and hip-width apart, with your hands on your hips. Tense the muscles on the front of your back hip as you lean forward, bending your front knee to stretch your hip flexors.

Technique tips
Make the movement nice and smooth, without trying to go too far. A variation of this stretch is to join the stretches up into a kind of forward "walking stretch," stretching one side, stepping forward and then stretching the other rather than returning to the beginning position after each rep.

Suggested number of reps in one set
7–10 on each side.

22. PULLING KNEES TO CHEST

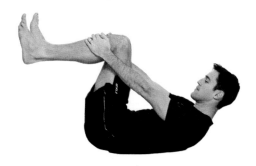 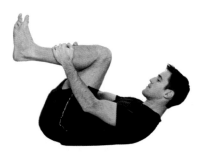

Main area and muscles stretched
Stretches the hip flexors.

Technique
Lie on your back, with your knees bent and your hands high up on your shins (toward, but not on, your knees). Push both shins away from your body to engage your muscles, and then smoothly pull both legs back toward your body.

Technique tips
If the above is too hard to do with both legs at once, do one at a time, still using both hands to stretch. Have a cushion behind your head if it helps to prevent your neck and shoulders from becoming tense.

Suggested number of reps in one set
7–10.

23. KNEELING UP QUAD STRETCH

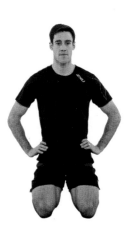 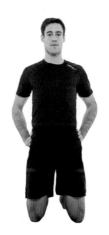 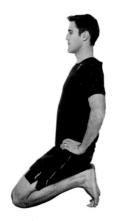
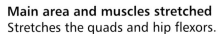
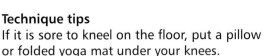

Main area and muscles stretched
Stretches the quads and hip flexors.

Technique
Sit on your heels with your hands on your hips. As you continuously tense the front of your hips and your lower abdomen, sit up and push your hips forward to stretch your quads and hip flexors. Make it an even stronger stretch by tensing your chest and then drawing your shoulders back at the same time as you push your hips forward.

Technique tips
If it is sore to kneel on the floor, put a pillow or folded yoga mat under your knees.

Suggested number of reps in one set
7–10.

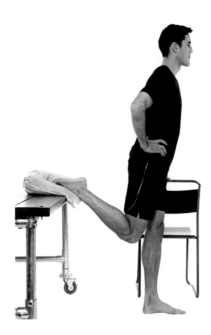
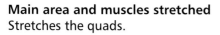
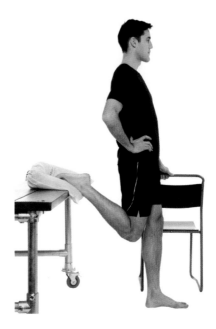

Main area and muscles stretched
Stretches the quads.

Technique
Rest your foot behind you on a table with padding under your foot, or on the back or arm of a sofa. Push the foot of your bent leg backward behind you (never downward) into the table or sofa continuously as you move your hips as far forward and then as far back toward your back foot as you can comfortably do, without pushing beyond any discomfort. Hold onto something so that you are stable and to keep your knee steady and straight as you stretch, stopping it from wobbling from side to side. Going forward and backward once counts as one rep.

Technique tips
Make sure that your standing leg is far enough away from the table so that you can move your hips forward as far as is comfortable. If you are using a table then you can use a folded yoga mat, cushion, or pillow to protect your foot. Also make sure that when you move backward you do not "sit" at your hips, but keep your torso and the thigh you are stretching in one straight line.

Many people want to put the place where their foot joins their ankle on the desk, but actually you should put your foot further down, roughly one third of the way up from the toes.

Suggested number of reps in one set
7–10 on each side.

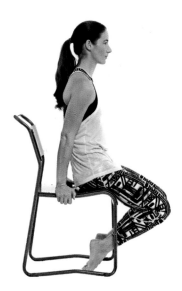
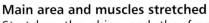
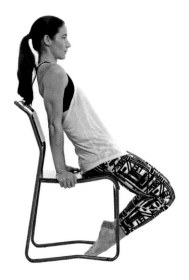

Main area and muscles stretched
Stretches the shins and the front of the ankles.

Technique
Sitting in a chair, tuck your feet underneath you with the tops of your feet on the floor. With your toes and feet continuously pushing down into floor, lean backward and forward to complete one rep.

Technique tips
If it is sore to have your toes tucked under try the Sitting Toe Stretch instead; it stretches your foot differently, but is very effective.

Suggested number of reps in one set
7–10.

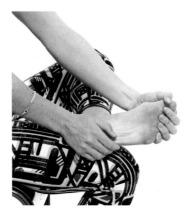

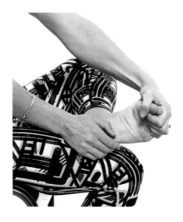

Main area and muscles stretched
Stretches the feet and toes.

Technique
Sit in a chair or on the floor and rest your foot on your leg. Hold your heel with your opposite hand to steady your foot and rest the hand of the same side on top of your foot, covering your toes. As your toes pull themselves upward continuously toward your knee, smoothly and gently push them down with the hand that is resting on top of them.

Technique tips
If you have tension or pain in your shins, only do this stretch if it does not cause any further pain or tension and try not to tense the shins as your toes pull themselves up.

If the joints crack a couple of times this is fine, but we do not try to make it happen. As usual, do not push through any pain.

Suggested number of reps in one set
7–10 on each side.

27. "CLAW" FOOT STRETCH

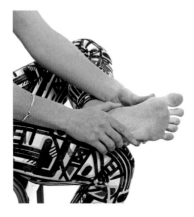

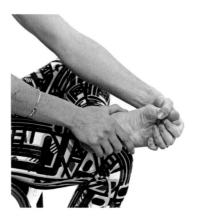

Main area and muscles stretched
Stretches the feet and toes.

Technique
Sit comfortably with your foot resting on your leg as you sit in a chair or on the floor. Tense your feet and toes by pushing your toes as far apart as you can. Then squeeze your foot with one hand, squeezing your toes back together. Release easily and then repeat.

Technique tips
The key is to keep the tension in your whole foot as you squeeze it.

Suggested number of reps in one set
7–10 on each foot.

Back of the Body

These stretches are for the back of your neck, torso, arms and legs. Please note that even though these stretches are great for the back, if you do have any issues with your back, neck, or elsewhere in the body please consult with your doctor or other healthcare provider before stretching.

Stretching the back of your body can make you feel taller, more energized, more stable on your feet, and, of course, more flexible.

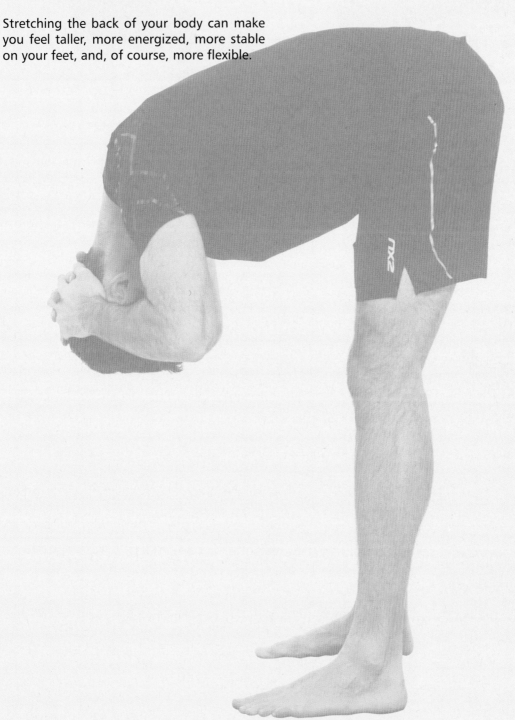

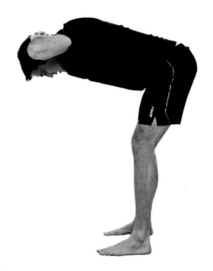
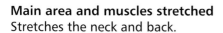
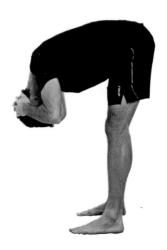

Main area and muscles stretched
Stretches the neck and back.

Technique
Stand with your feet shoulder-width apart, bent forward at the waist. Raise yourself slightly, with your hands clasped behind your head. As you look back up with your head and tense your back and hamstrings, pull your head down and lean down toward your knees against that resistance. Do not push through any pain and do not tense your muscles too strongly.

Technique tips
Make sure that you bend your knees and come up slowly out of this stretch to avoid dizziness. Don't put any weight on your head with your arms as you come up.

This stretch is great because it simultaneously stretches the neck, back and hamstrings. The key is to stay balanced and to have something sturdy to lean on in case of losing your balance.

Suggested number of reps in one set
5–7.

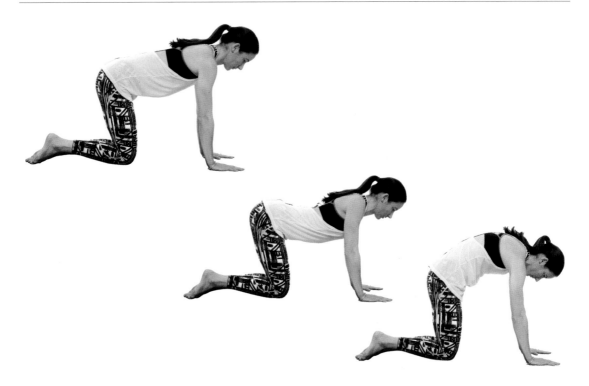

Main area and muscles stretched
Stretches the whole back.

Technique
Get onto your hands and knees and tense your back as you push it down, lowering your belly button toward the floor. Then keep the tension on as you arch your back up as far as you can go. From there you can push your back all the way down again and move fluidly from one to the other. Lowering and raising your back once counts as one rep.

Technique tips
Do not push through any pain and also remember to look up when your back is down, and to look down when your back is up.

Suggested number of reps in one set
7–10.

3. CHILD'S POSE WITH RESISTANCE

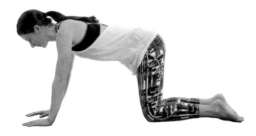
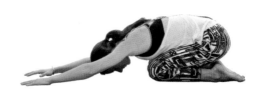

Main area and muscles stretched
Stretches the upper back and upper arms.

Technique
Get onto your hands and knees and, keeping a slight bend in your elbows, pull back and down into the ground with your hands. As you continuously pull down into the ground and back toward you, smoothly sit back on your heels. Return easily to the starting position and repeat.

Technique tips
If it is too easy then move your hands further forward and if it is too difficult, move your hands a little closer to your knees.

Suggested number of reps in one set
7–10.

4. ALL FOURS ARM OUT STRETCH

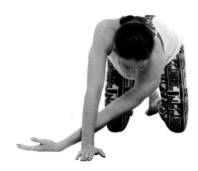
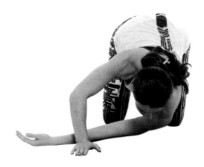

Main area and muscles stretched
Stretches the back of the arms and the shoulders.

Technique
Get down onto all fours and then lay one of your arms under your body pointing out to the other side, with the back of your hand on the floor. Push that hand down into the floor and bend your other arm to lower yourself and stretch the outside of your lower arm and shoulder.

Technique tips
If you tense the whole of your torso you will probably also be able to feel the stretch across the side of your body, adding extra benefits to the stretch.

Suggested number of reps in one set
7–10 on each side.

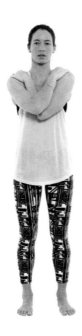
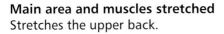
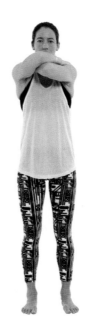

Main area and muscles stretched
Stretches the upper back.

Technique
Bend one of your arms in front of you and then place your other arm bent on top of it, so the elbows are one above the other. Do not let your arms cross over (they do in the photo—my mistake!), but have the hand of the upper arm on the shoulder and the hand of the lower arm lower down, just underneath the opposite shoulder. Squeezing your elbows together continuously move your elbows up and then down to stretch your shoulders and completing one rep.

Technique tips
You may not feel much happening in this stretch until after it is over. Try to keep the tension going between your shoulder blades as well to make the stretch even stronger. Swap which arm is on top halfway through.

Suggested number of reps in one set
7–10.

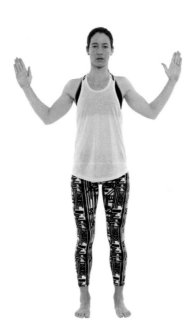

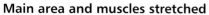

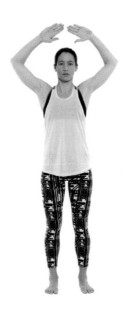

Main area and muscles stretched

Stretches the upper back and especially around the shoulder blades.

Technique

Raise your arms and have them bent at your sides so that your elbows are a little lower than your shoulders. Tensing the muscles of your shoulders and upper back move your arms around and up in a smooth arc, hands meeting and then overlapping above your head and down again smoothly to complete one rep.

Technique tips

This stretch certainly lets you know if you have any sticking points or restrictions around your shoulder blades. If you can feel certain areas that do not move easily and there is no pain, then persist with this stretch to improve it. Do be careful if you have an existing or previous shoulder injury.

Suggested number of reps in one set

7–10.

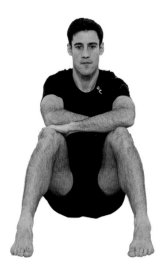
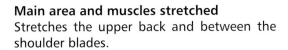
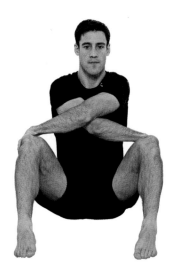

Main area and muscles stretched
Stretches the upper back and between the shoulder blades.

Technique
Sit with your knees bent in front of you and crossing your arms at the elbows, place a hand on each knee. Tensing the muscles of your arms, shoulders and upper back, slowly pull out against that resistance with your knees as far as you can go comfortably and then return easily and repeat.

Technique tips
Maintain constant tension in your arms and between your shoulder blades and switch which arm is on top half way through your set.

Suggested number of reps in one set
7–10.

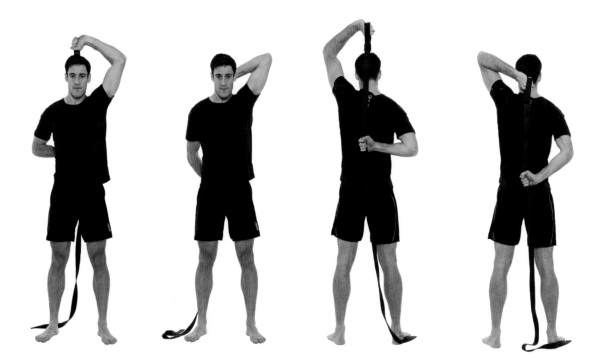

Main area and muscles stretched

Stretches the triceps and the side of the torso.

Technique

Hold a yoga strap or belt in your hand and put that hand behind your head. Lift your other hand up behind your back to grasp the strap as high up as you can.

Holding the strap firmly, tense your muscles by pulling your upper arm upward and as it keeps pulling up, allow the lower arm to pull it smoothly downward to stretch it. Only pull it down as far as you can go comfortably. One up and downward movement is one rep.

Technique tips

In case this is confusing you can think of it this way; the upper arm always pulls up, the lower arm always pulls down, but the lower arm always wins. When you have pulled the upper arm as far down as is comfortable, relax and return it up to the starting position.

Suggested number of reps in one set

7–10 on each side.

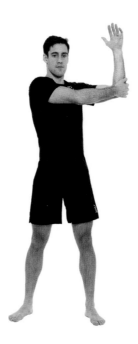

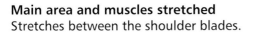

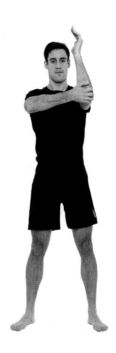

Main area and muscles stretched
Stretches between the shoulder blades.

Technique
Have your arm bent at a right angle and out beside you, your elbow level with your shoulder. Hold the outside of your bent arm at the elbow with your opposite hand.

As your bent arm pulls out and behind you continuously, pull it smoothly toward the midline of your body as far as it will go comfortably.

Technique tips
Do not pull through any pain and keep the movement nice and smooth.

Suggested number of reps in one set
7–10 on each side.

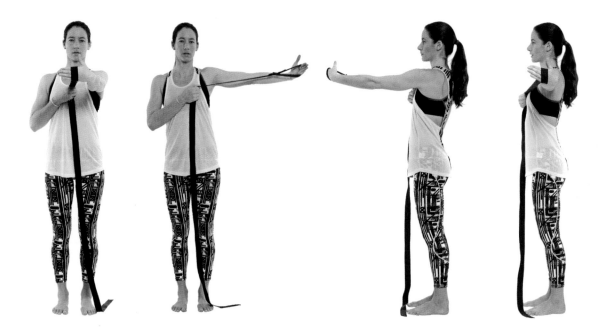

Main area and muscles stretched

Stretches the forearm, wrist and back of the hand.

Technique

Create a loop in your yoga strap and put your hand into the loop. Move your hand in front of your body, with your arm straight, holding the yoga strap with the other hand, which is in front of your chest. As your hand pushes outward into the strap continuously, smoothly move your hand out in an arc out to the side, stretching your forearm.

Technique tips

The strap will have to lengthen slightly a little as your arm moves out, so you can either pay it out a little (in which case you need to make sure it is still tight enough so that you still to get a stretch all the way through the movement) or you can move the hand that is holding the strap accordingly.

Suggested number of reps in one set

7–10 on each side.

11. BENDING WRIST DOWN

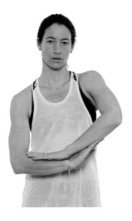 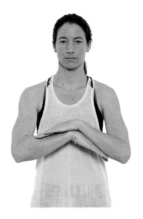

Main area and muscles stretched
Stretches the forearm and wrist.

Technique
Have one arm in front of you, palm facing down. Then bend that arm at the wrist, so that your hand is sloping up. Rest your other arm on top of that arm, keeping the lower wrist bent, one wrist on top of the other. Grasp the lower arm with the upper hand and pushing the lower hand continuously up into the arm on top, bend your upper arm downward to stretch the lower wrist.

Technique tips
Try to keep your shoulders down and relaxed as you do this stretch. You do not need to hold onto your lower arm; some people prefer to in order to get extra leverage, but others prefer not to, either way is fine.

Suggested number of reps in one set
7–10 on each side.

12. FINGER INTERLINKED STRETCH

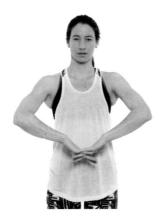 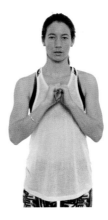

Main area and muscles stretched
Stretches the fingers and the back of the forearms.

Technique
Interlink your fingers, with them pointing in and down instead of out. Keeping your hands and fingers straight, tense your fingers and hands continuously as you gently pull your palms together to stretch your fingers and forearms.

Technique tips
Do not tense your muscles very hard to begin with, but build the intensity slowly in order to warm up.

Suggested number of reps in one set
6–7.

13. LAT STRETCH AT DESK

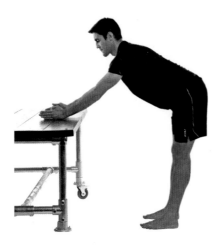 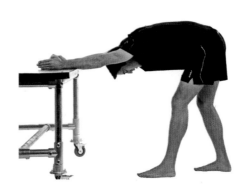

Main area and muscles stretched
Stretches the lats and upper back.

Technique
Put your hands down on a desk, parallel, on their sides and facing each other, about one hand span apart.

Whilst continuously pulling your hands down into the desk, step back with one foot and lower your torso toward the floor, keeping your arms straight. Only go as far as you can comfortably and then return easily to the starting position.

Technique tips
Do not lean forward onto your hands, but keep all the weight on your front leg. The key is to move smoothly away from the table as you go down, in order to feel a lengthening in the back and shoulders as you stretch. Keep pulling down into the table continuously. Also, do not worry if you cannot lower your torso until it is parallel with the floor, just go as far as you can without discomfort.

Suggested number of reps in one set
7–10.

14. CROSS OVER LEG PULL IN STRETCH

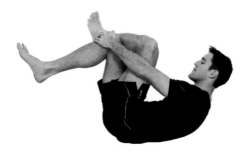 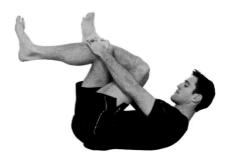

Main area and muscles stretched
Stretches the backs of the thighs and hips.

Technique
Lying on your back with one leg crossed over the other, link your hands around your lower knee. That knee pushes itself away from your body continuously as you pull your legs back toward your body together, with your arms, to stretch.

Technique tips
This stretches both legs at once, but in different ways, so it is important to stretch both sides.

Suggested number of reps in one set
7–10 on each side.

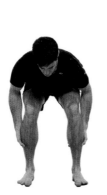 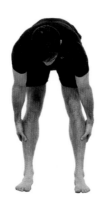 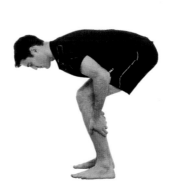 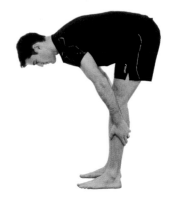

Main area and muscles stretched
Stretches the central hamstrings.

Technique
Standing with your feet shoulder-width apart and bent over at the waist, bend your knees and tense the backs of your legs. Keep your legs tense as you smoothly stick your bottom up in the air, straightening your legs to stretch your hamstrings. Squatting down and up again is one rep. Before you come up out of the stretch, engage your abdominal muscles and bend your knees, to avoid straining your lower back.

Technique tips
Do not worry if you cannot go very far down or up, focus on maintaining the tension as you move and you will get a good stretch.

Suggested number of reps in one set
7–10 reps.

16. SQUAT TO HAMSTRING STRETCH

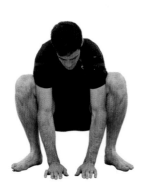 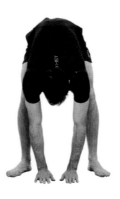 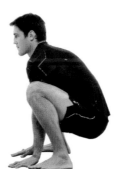 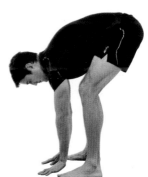

Main area and muscles stretched
Stretches the central hamstrings.

Technique
Sit in a deep squatting pose, tense the backs of your legs and smoothly lift your bottom up into air to stretch your hamstrings. As you push your bottom up, maintain the tension in the backs of the legs. Relax down to the starting position and repeat.

Technique tips
Don't worry if your heels are not on the floor, or if you need to hold onto something sturdy to stabilize you. Only go as high as you can comfortably go.

Suggested number of reps in one set
7–10.

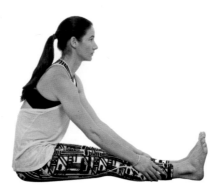

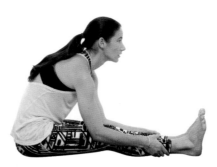

Main area and muscles stretched
Stretches the hamstrings.

Technique
Sit comfortably with your legs out in front of you, slightly bent, and your feet close together but not touching. Pull your feet down into the ground continuously as you smoothly lean forward from your hips as far as you can go comfortably. It is fine to grasp behind your knees, your calves or ankles if you can't reach your feet.

Technique tips
Don't worry if you can't go very far, try not to compensate by bending your back.

Suggested number of reps in one set
7–10.

18. KNEELING SIT BACK

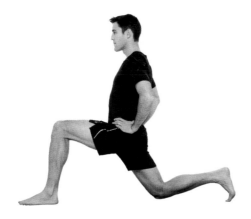 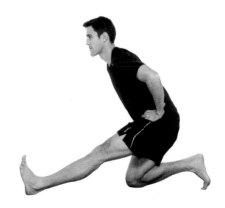

Main area and muscles stretched
Stretches the hamstrings.

Technique
Kneel down on one knee, your other leg bent in front of you with the foot slightly further forward than it would naturally be. Start with your front knee very bent and as the front foot pulls continuously down into the ground, sit back smoothly to stretch the back of that leg.

Technique tips
If it is sore to kneel on the floor, put some padding under your knee. Remember that the front foot is pulling down and into the floor and as you come back the toes should point to the sky.

Suggested number of reps in one set
7–10 on each side.

19. STRAIGHT LEG LEAN FORWARD

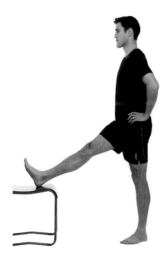 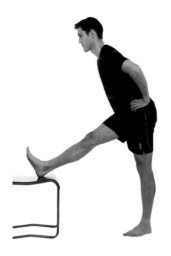

Main area and muscles stretched
Stretches the hamstrings.

Technique
Stand with your leg up on a low wall, desk, or chair, with a slight bend in your knee. Pulling your foot downward constantly, smoothly lean forward from your hips to stretch the back of that leg. Make sure that you are not transferring your weight forward onto your leg that is raised, but keep your weight on your standing leg.

Technique tips
Do not go further than it is comfortable to go, as in the long term this may create more tightness in your hamstrings.

Suggested number of reps in one set
7–10 on each side.

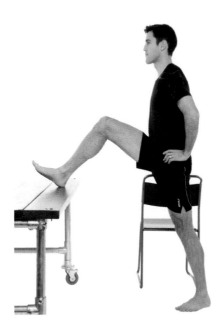 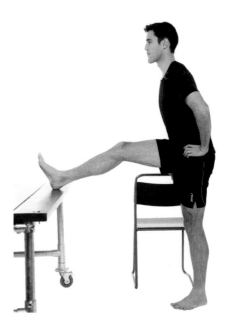

Main area and muscles stretched
Stretches the central hamstrings mainly.

Technique
Stand with one foot out in front of you on a table, step, or other secure surface. Bend the upper leg's knee as much as possible, and while you continuously pull that foot down and back into the table (with the toes pointing up as much as is comfortable), smoothly lengthen your leg by sticking your bottom out behind you.

Technique tips
Make sure that you start with your leg as bent as you can and start pulling back with your foot in that position, otherwise you will miss the opportunity to stretch through the whole range of motion. Do not put any of your body's weight on your bent leg, only on your standing leg. Do not straighten your leg completely, but only go as far as is comfortable so that you can maintain the tension in your muscles.

Suggested number of reps in one set
7–10 on each side.

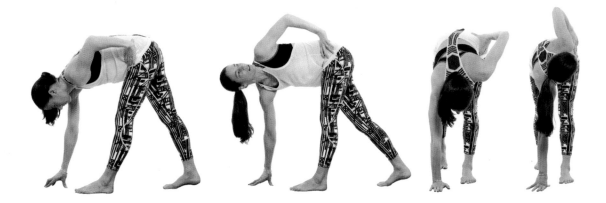

Main area and muscles stretched
Stretches the lateral hamstrings.

Technique
Bend over from the hips and transfer all of your weight onto one leg. That leg should be fairly straight with only a slight bend in the knee and your other leg should be behind you, slightly bent and relaxed. Bend your front knee and then push that foot down into the ground to tense the outside/ back of your leg. Then smoothly stick your bottom up into the air on that side only to stretch. Bend your knee again to return to the starting position and repeat.

Pushing your hip up and down again once is one rep.

Technique tips
The key is to let the hip of the back leg drop down and stay relaxed, and make the front leg do all of the work. Also be careful not to twist your hips backward or forward, but only up into the air on the side you are stretching, pushing that hip up. It may be a good idea to have something sturdy beside you to hold onto.

Suggested number of reps in one set
7–10 on each side.

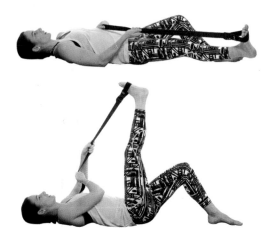
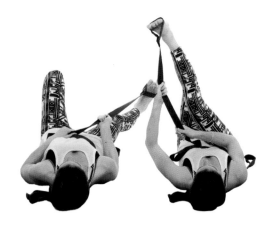

Main area and muscles stretched
Stretches the lateral hamstrings and glutes.

Technique
Stretch the outside/back of your thighs (lateral hamstrings) by lying down and putting the loop of a strap around one foot. Starting with the leg of that foot down and out to the side, it pulls down and outward while you pull it up and across your body, toward the opposite shoulder with the yoga strap. The leg being pulled up and relaxing back again down once counts as one rep.

Technique tips
Try not to pull your leg down towards the body with the strap, but up and across the body, so you are pulling up/ parallel to the floor. This helps us not to compress the hip joint. Keep the leg you are stretching straight throughout the movement and only go as far as you can comfortably go.

Suggested number of reps in one set
7–10 on each side.

23. HEEL DROP STRETCH

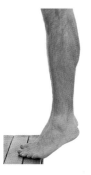
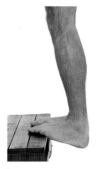

Main area and muscles stretched
Stretches the calves and Achilles tendon.

Technique
Stand with the balls of your feet on the edge of a step, a little closer than shoulder-width apart, heels hanging off. Hold onto something sturdy for balance throughout the stretch. Tense your calves as you lower yourself slowly, stretching out your calves and Achilles. If this stretch is too hard to do with resistance, then do one leg at a time, alternating between them.

Technique tips
You will most likely need to let your heels get down to the level of the step or just below, to be able to engage the muscle without blocking the movement altogether. Return quickly and easily to the starting position when you have gone as far as you can comfortably.

Suggested number of reps in one set
5–7.

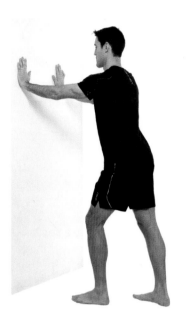 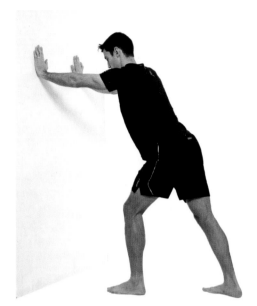 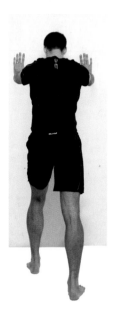

Main area and muscles stretched
Stretches the calves.

Technique
Stand facing a wall with one foot quite a bit further back than the other. As you push the toes of your back foot down into the ground, push your arms forward into the wall, pushing your back heel down against resistance.

Rock the front knee backward and forward to create movement in the stretch. The front knee moving forward and backward once is one rep.

Technique tips
There are variations of this stretch in the outside and inside of the leg sections in case you would like to stretch a different area of your calf.

Suggested number of reps in one set
7–10 on each side.

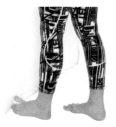 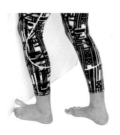 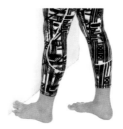 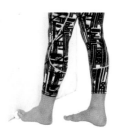

Main area and muscles stretched
Stretches the feet.

Technique
Place a golf ball in the angle where the wall and the floor meet. Position your big and second toe on the golf ball and rest your foot on the floor in that position. Have your other foot fairly far behind you, only as far as is comfortable. Push your toes into the golf ball as you lean forward to stretch your toes and foot.

Change this exercise by placing the golf ball under your middle toes, and then again with the golf ball under your fourth and little toes.

Technique tips
If this exercise is painful in your feet at all then do not push down as hard with your toes, or lean as far forward. If you do not get much of a stretch, then try putting the golf ball against a step instead of a wall, so that you can lean further forward over it.

Suggested number of reps in one set
2–3 with the golf ball in each position, on each side.

26. SITTING TOE STRETCH

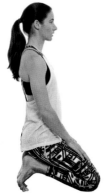 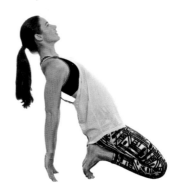

Main area and muscles stretched
Stretches the soles of the feet and the toes.

Technique
Sit on your heels, with your toes tucked underneath your feet. Push your toes down into the ground as you lean back and then forward to stretch the soles of your feet and toes. Rocking backward and forward once is one rep.

(If you change this stretch by having your toes and feet flat on the ground, you can stretch the front of your ankles and shins. If you do not feel a stretch then you can raise your toes by placing a towel or small cushion underneath the top part of your foot and your toes, and try again.)

Technique tips
The key to this stretch is to maintain the tension by having the toes push themselves down into the floor continuously.

Suggested number of reps in one set
5–7.

Outside of the Body

These stretches are for the outside of the neck, torso, legs, and ankles. We do not often think about the sides of our bodies, unless they are painful, but tightness in these areas can pull us out of alignment very strongly.

Stretching the outside of the body helps to create much more freedom and ease of movement.

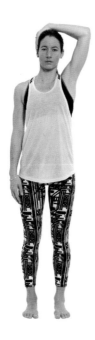

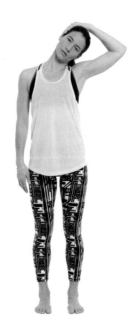

Main area and muscles stretched
Stretches the side of the neck.

Technique
Moderately tense your neck and then use your opposite hand to pull your head down smoothly toward the shoulder of that arm. Make the movement smoothly and gently and only go as far as you can comfortably.

When you return from the first rep, you can move your head further towards the other shoulder and start the stretch from there. Continue to do this for each subsequent stretch.

When coming back to the starting position do not weigh your head down with your arm at all, but let it return very easily.

Technique tips
The key to this stretch is to do it gently, to create the tension in the neck before you move it at all and do not try to make your neck click at all (although it may do so naturally by itself, which is fine). Be careful if you have neck problems and do not push through any pain.

Suggested number of reps in one set
3–5 on each side.

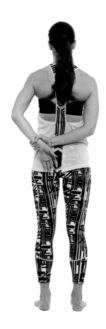
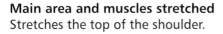
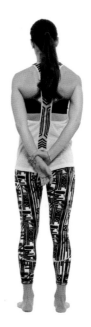

Main area and muscles stretched
Stretches the top of the shoulder.

Technique
With your arms behind your back, grasp one wrist and have the elbow of that arm bent. The bent elbow pulls itself upwards and out to the side as the other arm pulls it diagonally back down towards the opposite foot to stretch the top of the shoulder.

Technique tips
Try to keep the shoulders down and do not tense the neck as you stretch. Be careful if you have shoulder problems and do not push through any pain.

Suggested number of reps in one set
5–7 on each side.

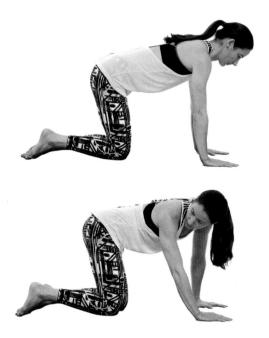

Main area and muscles stretched
Stretches the back and the sides of the torso.

Technique
Get into position on your hands and knees, with your back flat. Tense your back and sides and move your head around to look down your left side, and curve your hips to the left and toward your head, curling yourself like a letter 'C'. Come back to the starting position easily and then repeat on the other side.

Technique tips
Try not to turn your head, but keep looking down so that your ear is moving closer to your hips rather than your chin.

Suggested number of reps in one set
7–10 on each side.

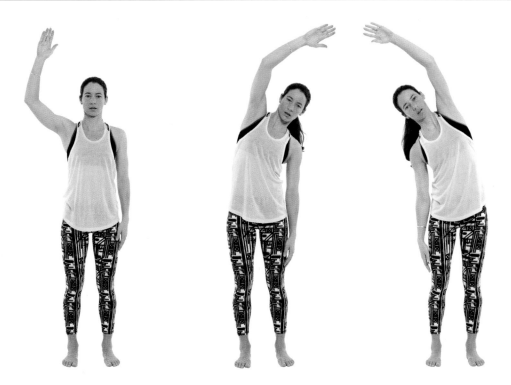

Main area and muscles stretched
Stretches the sides of your torso.

Technique
Standing with your feet shoulder-width apart rest one hand on your hip. Raise your other hand above your head, keeping it slightly bent and out to the side. Then, tensing the muscles of that side push your arm over your head as you lean sideways. Return easily to the start before switching arms and repeating on the other side.

Technique tips
Try not to twist forward or backward, which often occurs as the body tries to avoid tight areas.

Although the model above does not have her hand on her hip, it is best to do so if you feel better with that support. However, you can also do it without if it does not compromise your technique.

Suggested number of reps in one set
7–10 on each side.

5. ABDUCTOR BENT LEG STRETCH

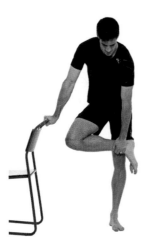 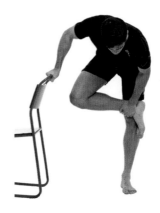

Main area and muscles stretched
Stretches the glutes and iliotibial band (ITB).

Technique
Stand on one leg, the other leg bent across it, its ankle just above your standing leg's knee. Hold it in place with your opposite hand. As your bent leg continuously pushes backward into your standing leg, lean forward smoothly to stretch the glutes and ITB of your bent leg.

Technique tips
It is best to lean on a chair, desk, or wall for stability.

Suggested number of reps in one set
7–10 on each side.

6. LEAN OVER BENT KNEE

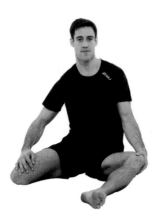 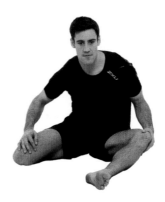

Main area and muscles stretched
Stretches the abductors.

Technique
Sit with your leg bent in front of you, with your knee at a greater than 90° angle and your other leg bent out to the side. Support your knee with your hand or a block or cushion. The knee pushes down continuously into your hand as you lean forward to stretch the abductors and glutes. After leaning forward smoothly as far as you can comfortably go, return easily to the starting position.

Technique tips
Try not to bend your spine very much as you lean forward as this will not help your stretch.

If you are a bit tight and find yourself falling over to the side, you can use your opposite hand to support your knee and your hand on the same side to balance with.

Suggested number of reps in one set
7–10 on each side.

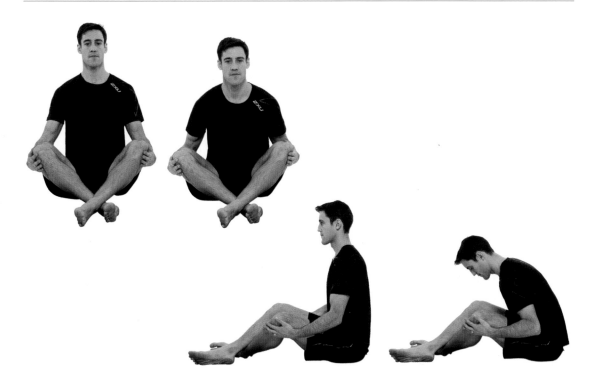

Main area and muscles stretched
The back of your hips and outside of your thighs.

Technique
Sit comfortably with your legs crossed and then uncross them a bit so that your legs are crossed at your calves in front of you. Support your knees with your hands.

Create tension in your abductors by having your knees push down into your hands and feet push themselves down toward the ground. Maintaining that continuous tension, gently and smoothly lean forward, without straining. Do not hold the stretch, but return easily to the start and then repeat.

After several reps, swap your legs round (place the lower one on top instead) and repeat. Leaning forward and backward once is one rep.

Technique tips
This stretch looks deceptively easily until you try it. Resistance is definitely the magic ingredient, transforming a normally easy movement into a challenging stretch for many. Keep your lower back straight throughout the stretch.

Suggested number of reps in one set
5–7.

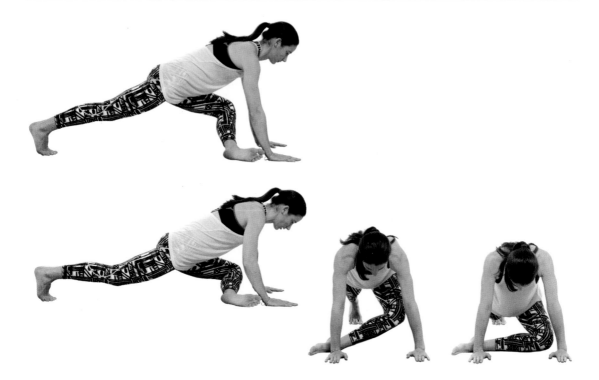

Main area and muscles stretched
Stretches the abductors.

Technique
Get into a push-up position and bend one leg in front of you (but behind your hands), so that your lower leg is perpendicular to your body, with its knee in the air, and that foot pushing down into the ground. Do a push-up over your front leg, and as your hips move downwards your knee will also move down, stretching your abductors. Only go as far down as you can comfortably and return easily.

Technique tips
This is quite a hard stretch, which you can also do kneeling on your back leg to make it easier. Do not worry if you can only manage a small movement, it is more important to stay within a comfortable range. Some people confuse this with pigeon stretch in yoga, but it is important that you have the leg perpendicular and your knee in the air.

Some people's knees will touch the floor at the end of the stretch, and some will not. Only go as far as you can comfortably and if you have knee issues then start with an easier stretch.

Suggested number of reps in one set
7–10 on each side.

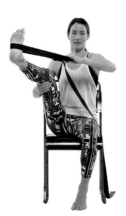
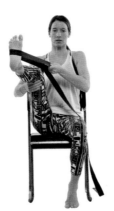

Main area and muscles stretched
Stretches the abductors.

Technique
Sit in a chair and make a loop with a yoga strap or towel. Have one leg in the air, bent at 90°, swung to the outside, with the hand of the same side holding the leg under the knee to stabilize it. Place the loop around the foot and swing it out as far as you can, and then using the strap pull your foot in toward the opposite shoulder smoothly.

Technique tips
It is important to keep the knee in the same position, so that it does not swing out with your foot.

Suggested number of reps in one set
5–7 on each side.

10. PULL BENT LEG TOWARD YOU

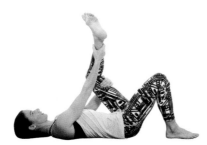
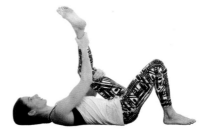

Main area and muscles stretched
Stretches the abductors.

Technique
With your leg raised in the air and the knee at a greater than 90° angle, hold it with your hands as shown. As it continuously pushes away from you, let it go as far as you can reach and then pull it back toward your head. Return to the starting position and repeat.

Technique tips
The trick with this stretch is to keep the knee at the same angle when you pull it back and not to bend it more. You also want to be able to see inside of the leg all the way through, rather than the top of it, as it is rotated outwards all the way through.

You can use a pillow to prevent your neck from tensing up if that helps.

Suggested number of reps in one set
5-7 on each side.

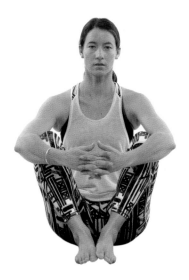
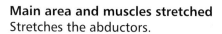
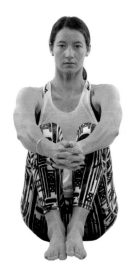

Main area and muscles stretched
Stretches the abductors.

Technique
Sitting with your knees bent in front of chest and your feet together, place your arms around your legs and clasp your hands. As your knees push out continuously, your arms straighten and squeeze in to stretch your abductors. Return easily to the start and repeat. The knees moving together and out again once is one rep.

Technique tips
Keep your shoulders down throughout the movement and do not tense your neck or shoulders.

Suggested number of reps in one set
5–7.

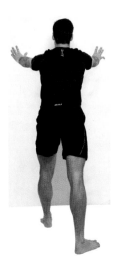

Main area and muscles stretched
Stretches the outside of the calf.

Technique
Get into a calf stretch position with one foot behind you and one bent in front as you push into a wall. However before you move, turn your back foot outward instead of straight forward. Push the toes of that foot into the floor and then bend your front knee more to stretch, keeping your back leg straight. Return easily to the start position and repeat.

Technique tips
You can play around with the angle until you feel a stretch. To make it stronger have your back foot further away and to make it easier have your back foot closer to the wall.

Some people get a better stretch by turning their foot inwards instead, and others by turning it outwards. Experiment to see which gets you the best stretch for your outer calf.

Suggested number of reps in one set
5–7 on each side.

13. OUTER ANKLE STRETCH

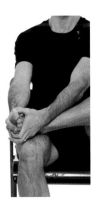 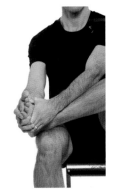

Main area and muscles stretched
Stretches the outside of the ankle.

Technique
Sitting with one leg across the other, hold your foot with both hands, which pushes itself away from you and down toes first. Keeping your ankle still, pull your foot back up and toward you smoothly with your hands.

Technique tips
Please note that your leg and ankle do not move position in this stretch (although they will turn a little), the stretch depends on rotating your foot at the ankle.

Suggested number of reps in one set
5–7 on each side.

Inside of the Legs

This is the smallest section, but definitely not the least important! Stretching your inner legs can have huge benefits on the alignment of your whole body. They do especially like to be warmed up, so never go in really hard right away, but stretch them more gently with less resistance and then build the resistance and intensity slowly.

Stretching the inside of your legs and your groin can make you feel released all the way up through the midline of your body. It can also make you feel more open and "in your center of gravity" at the same time.

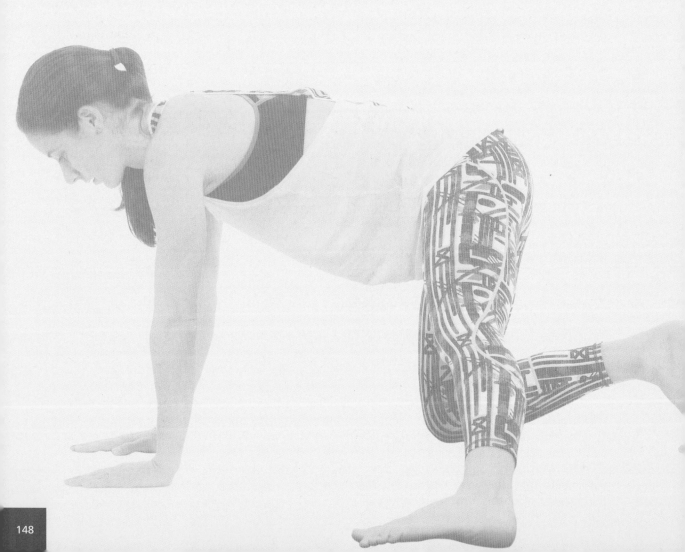

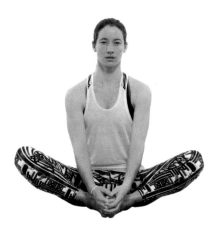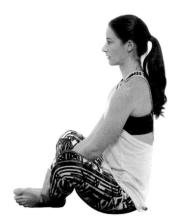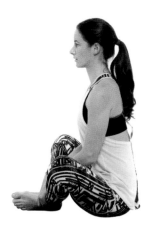

Main area and muscles stretched
Stretches the groin.

Technique
This is a strong stretch although it does not look like much from the outside. Sit with your feet together, holding your ankles and resting your arms on your legs. Your legs push up into your arms and your arms push down into your legs, but neither move, in order to create the resistance for the stretch, as you rock your hips forward to stretch your groin.

You return by relaxing backwards and repeat the stretch by rocking forwards again.

Technique tips
If this is hard to understand pretend that you have something in front of your abdomen and then try to push it forward with your hip bones. Try not to lean forward with your back, but concentrate on only shifting the hips forward. Continuing to hold onto your legs as you pull backward with your hands can help you to rock your hips forward.

Suggested number of reps in one set
7–10.

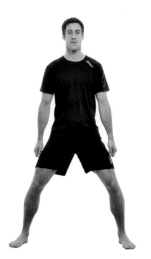 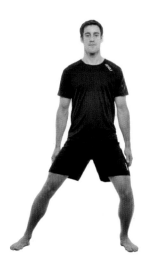 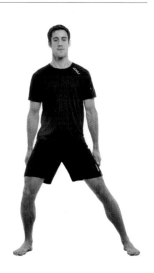

Main area and muscles stretched
Stretches the adductors.

Technique
Squat, with your hips tucked underneath you, pulling your feet together into the floor (they don't move, they just pull into the floor without rolling the knees inward).

Maintain that tension on the inside of the legs by squeezing the feet together and slide to one side to stretch the inside (adductors) of the leg that is becoming straighter. Be careful not to raise your hips, but slide evenly as if your bottom is moving along a shelf. Slide back all the way to the other side. Sliding to one side and then the other counts as one rep.

Technique tips
It can be hard to keep your hips tucked under if you're not used to it. Imagine that you are trying to flatten the curve in your lower back.

Suggested number of reps in one set
7–10.

3. SITTING BACK ADDUCTORS

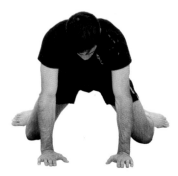 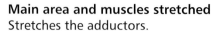 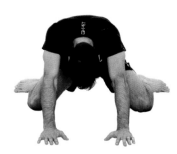

Main area and muscles stretched
Stretches the adductors.

Technique
On your hands and knees, place your knees even further apart and have your toes pointing outward as far as it is comfortable. Squeeze your knees into the floor and smoothly sit back. When you have gone as far as you can without discomfort, come back up to the starting position and repeat.

Technique tips
You may find that this is sore on your knees, in which case you can try putting padding underneath them, but if that does not help try an alternative stretch.

Suggested number of reps in one set
7–10.

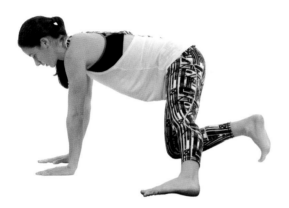
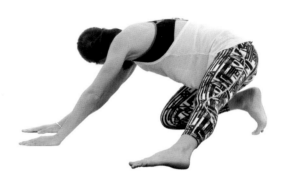

Main area and muscles stretched
Stretches the adductors.

Technique
On your hands and knees put one leg out to the side, straight, with your foot pointing forward. Continuously pull your foot down into the ground and slightly toward you as you sit back to stretch the adductors of your straight leg. Then return easily to the start position.

Technique tips
If your knee is sore on the floor, put some padding underneath it. Intensify the stretch by rolling your torso away from the leg you are stretching and looking away from your straight leg.

Suggested number of reps in one set
7–10 on each side.

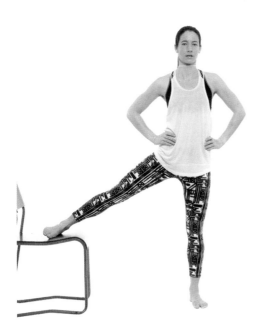
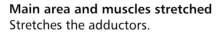
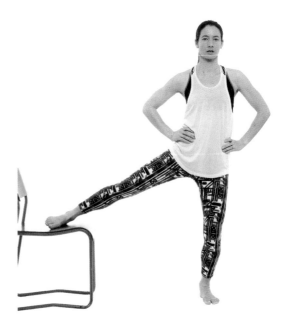

Main area and muscles stretched
Stretches the adductors.

Technique
With your foot up on a chair straight out to one side, keep that leg straight and pull the foot down into the chair continuously to engage the adductors of that leg. Keeping that force on, smoothly bend your standing leg as far as you can comfortably to stretch the adductors of the leg out to the side and then return easily to the starting position. Bending and straightening the knee of your standing leg once counts as one rep.

Technique tips
Start with your standing leg straight and your center of gravity over that leg. If you need to hold onto something to maintain your balance please do so. Make sure that you move smoothly and do not rush the movement. Also do not bend forward from the hips as you bend your standing leg.

Suggested number of reps in one set
7–10 on each side.

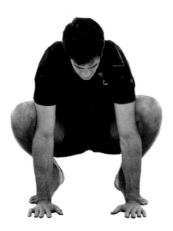 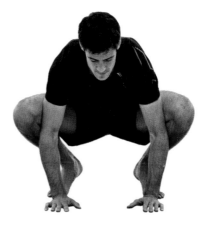

Main area and muscles stretched
Stretches the adductors.

Technique
Sit in a squatting position and place your hands on the ground in front of you, with your arms resting against the inside of your legs. Lean forward and while you squeeze inward with your knees, push your knees apart steadily with your elbows, stretching your adductors. When you have gone as far as you can comfortably go, return easily to the starting position.

Technique tips
The aim of this stretch is not to balance on your arms, only to lean forward to let gravity and your weight help to open your legs.

Suggested number of reps in one set
7–10.

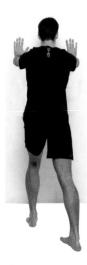

Main area and muscles stretched
Stretches the inside calves.

Technique
Stand facing a wall with one foot quite a bit further back than the other and turn your back foot inward. As you push the toes of your back foot down into the ground, push your arms forward into the wall, pushing your back heel down against resistance.

Move the front knee backward and forward to create movement in the stretch. The front knee moving forward and backward once is one rep.

Technique tips
There are variations of this stretch in the outside and back of the body sections in case you would like to stretch a different area of your calf.

Please note that some people find they get a better stretch on the inside of their calf by turning their foot out instead, and others prefer to do it as shown. I recommend you try both and see which way is best for you.

Suggested number of reps in one set
7–10 on each side.

8. INNER ANKLE STRETCH

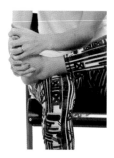
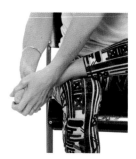

Main area and muscles stretched
Stretches the inside of the ankle.

Technique
Sitting with one leg across the other, hold your foot with both hands, as it pulls itself toward you. Keeping your ankle still, gently push your foot outwards again, stretching the inside of your ankle and foot. Let the foot return back up to the start easily, with no resistance, and repeat.

Technique tips
Please note that your leg and ankle do not move position in this stretch (although they will turn a little); it all comes from rotating your foot at the ankle.

Suggested number of reps in one set
5–7 on each side.

11 Moving Stretch Routines

These routines contain stretches that help you work toward a specific stretching goal. It is up to you how often you do a routine—you could do one routine every day for 30 days initially and thereafter for 5 or 6 days a week. Or you could cycle through all of the routines doing a different one on each day.

You can also create your own routine from the individual stretches and use these routines as a guideline. If you do want to create your own then I recommend starting with the stretches you find the most easy and building to the ones you find harder to do , with one or two more pleasant ones at the end. Generally speaking, it is better to include a mixture of upper and lower body stretches.

The number of reps that I suggest per set is given under each stretch. It is a suggested number because everyone's body is different and I recommend that you find what works best for you. If you are new to stretching then you can do one set of each stretch to start with and as you become more experienced you can do two to three sets of each stretch. Please go through the descriptions of the stretches before you try them and pay attention to the extra tips, which will help you to get the most out of each stretch.

You will notice that each routine is being demonstrated by a different person. Each of the eight models did their specific routine daily for 30 days (except one, who did two weeks due to illness) and we took before and after photos so that we could show how someone might benefit from each specific routine. All we asked them to do was to stand naturally in each picture and I promise that we did not ask them to stand taller in the after photos! We also measured their range of motion using the same flexibility tests in this book to see how the stretching affected it and these results are mentioned after each routine.

These models are all people I know personally to varying degrees, rather than fitness models, so we can call them "normal people," if there is such a thing. Most of them did not have a specific stretching practice beforehand, they are from a variety of backgrounds with different professions and exercise routines, and all experienced benefits from their stretching. As your body is unique you will probably get different changes to the models, so it is best to keep an open mind and see what happens.

I hope you enjoy them!

All Around Flexibility Booster

These stretches are great for people who need to start building flexibility in general, but can also be used as a great warm up to a stretching session. As several of the stretches are whole-body movements, it is also a good routine to use to help the body re-learn to function as a whole. Because many of us sit bent at the waist it is easy to lose this ability and become restricted in areas where we should be able to move freely. As you do these stretches bear in mind that the whole body is connected and try to create tension across a wide area to help facilitate this "reintegration" of your body.

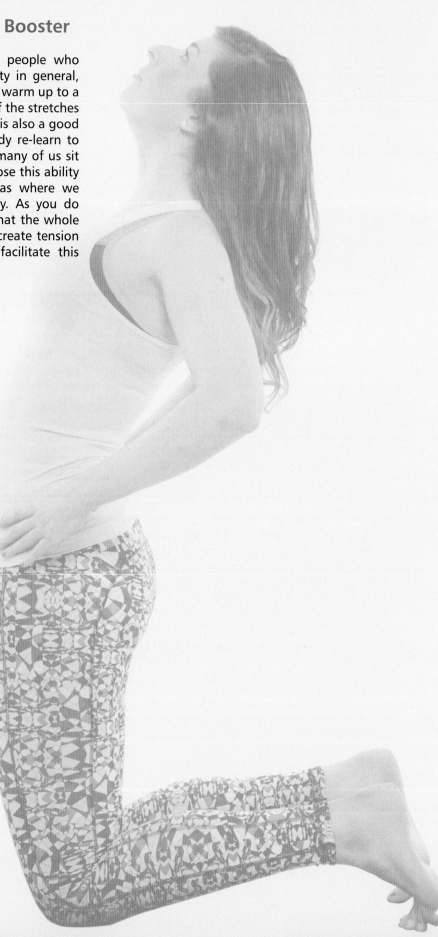

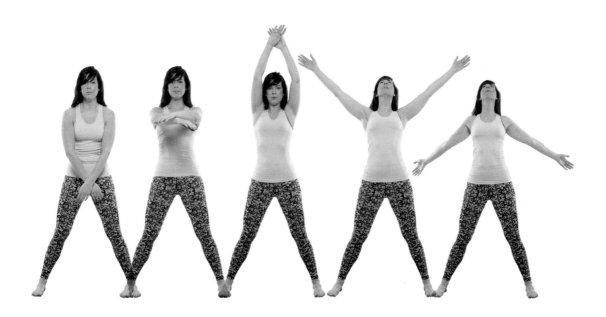

Main area and muscles stretched
Stretches the chest, shoulders, and hips.

Technique
Stand with your legs wide and your hands in front of your hips, crossed. Tense your chest, the front of your hips, and your arms and shoulders as you bring your arms up in front of your body and up over your head. When your hands are as far up above your head as they can go, separate them, bringing your arms out in a wide circle and slightly back behind you, leaning your head back and pushing your hips forward. Remember to keep your chest, shoulders and the front of your hips tense throughout the movement.

Come back to the starting position and repeat the movement, but with each circle outwards lead with a different finger for each rep—the forefinger, then middle finger, ring finger, then little finger, then thumb (with a very open hand) pushing out the most.

Technique tips
Only draw as wide a circle as you can comfortably do and do not push through any clunking in the shoulder or pain.

Suggested number of reps in one set
6 (1 initial one with the whole hand and then 1 with each finger).

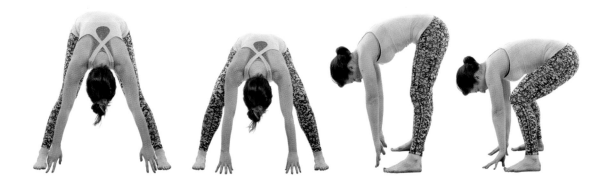

Main area and muscles stretched
Stretches the medial as well as central hamstrings.

Technique
Stand with your legs wide apart and bend forward from the hips and tense your abdominal muscles to protect your back. If you can reach the floor, then touch the floor, and if not then hold your calves. Tense the inside/back of your thighs by pulling your feet in together and backwards, but without moving your feet, and without rolling the knees inward.

Squat gently down to a comfortable level and then stick your bottom back up again, always tensing the inside back of your legs (medial hamstrings). One squat (down and up again) is one rep.

Technique tips
Do not worry if you cannot touch the floor or go down very far, just stay within a comfortable range and focus on moving against the resistance. The focus is not on what your posture looks like during this movement (although you do want to have good form), so much as the movement itself, which should be smooth, comfortable, and consistent.

Suggested number of reps in one set
7–10.

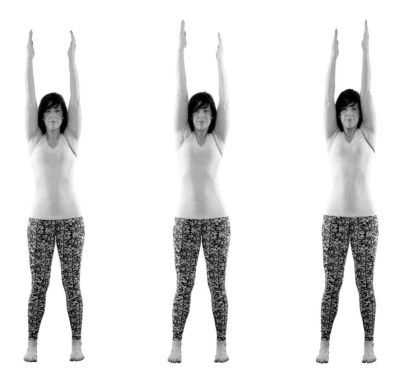

Main area and muscles stretched
Stretches the back and around your ribs.

Technique
Stand with your feet shoulder-width apart. Raise your hands out to the sides and up, and as you raise your hands imagine a line between them passing through your body. As the line passes up through your muscles, tense each muscle that it passes through.

With your hands above your head, parallel and facing each other, tense your whole torso and lift one hand up toward the sky, pushing as high as you can comfortably reach. Then let it return easily it to its starting position, keep the tension on in your muscles and push the other hand up toward the sky.

Technique tips
Make sure that your shoulders are as down and relaxed as they can be, except when being raised by the arm that is stretching. Try to be aware of your spine and ribs as you do this stretch and feel all of the muscles around them stretching.

Suggested number of reps in one set
7–10 on each side.

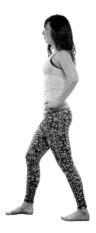 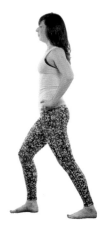

Main area and muscles stretched
Stretches the hip flexors.

Technique
Stand with one foot in front of the other and feet shoulder-width apart, with your hands on your hips. Tense the muscles on the front of your back hip as you push your hips forward, bending your knees to stretch your hip flexors.

Technique tips
Make the movement nice and smoothly, without trying to go too far.

You may need to adjust the distance between your feet to get the best stretch for you, having them further apart will lead to a stronger stretch and a closer together will lessen it.

Suggested number of reps in one set
7–10 on each side.

5. CENTRAL HAMSTRING SIT-BACK

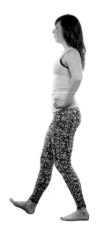 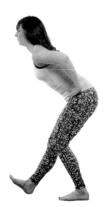

Main area and muscles stretched
Stretches the central hamstrings.

Technique
Stand comfortably with your feet fairly close and then step forward with one foot. Keep your front leg straight and as the front heel pulls back into the ground, sit back and bend forward from the hips simultaneously to stretch the central (middle) hamstring of that leg. Sitting back and then easily returning to the starting position counts as one rep.

Technique tips
Keep your the toes of your front foot pointed up toward the sky as much as you can comfortably do and make the movement as smoothly as you can. The knee of the other leg will bend naturally during the movement.

Suggested number of reps in one set
7–10 on each side.

6. ABDUCTOR BENT LEG STRETCH

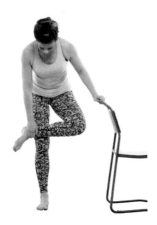

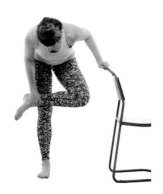

Main area and muscles stretched
Stretches the glutes and iliotibial band (ITB).

Technique
Stand with one leg bent across your other leg and its ankle above your standing leg's knee. Hold it in place with your opposite hand. As your bent leg continuously pushes backward into your standing leg, lean forward smoothly to stretch the glutes and ITB of your bent leg.

Technique tips
It is best to lean on a chair, desk, or wall for stability.

Suggested number of reps in one set
7–10 on each side.

7. KNEELING UP QUAD STRETCH

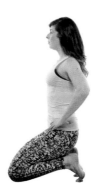

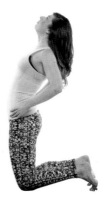

Main area and muscles stretched
Stretches the quads and hip flexors.

Technique
Sit on your heels with your hands on your hips. As you continuously tense the front of your hips and your lower abdomen, sit up and push your hips forward to stretch your quads and hip flexors. Make it an even stronger stretch by tensing your chest and then drawing your shoulders back at the same time as you push your hips forward.

Technique tips
If it is sore to kneel on the floor, put a pillow or folded yoga mat under your knees.

Suggested number of reps in one set
7–10.

Before

After

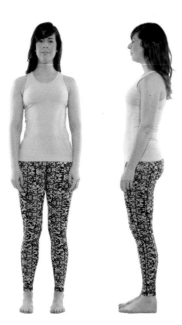

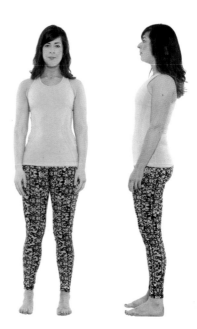

Katie added these stretches to her existing regular exercise routine (high-intensity cardio, body exercises and hockey) for a month and found that her performance in sport improved and she felt less tight and stiff. She particularly felt that these stretches were beneficial to her flexibility if she did them after a long or intense workout.

It is clear from the photos that Katie's posture has improved with her shoulders coming back, her head becoming more aligned and her neck longer and her hips opening. She also looks stronger and more secure in her balance. In the flexibility tests her range of motion improved by 1–3 inches across all of the tests bar one.

Freedom to Move

These stretches are great for people who want to free their bodies, feel looser and freer to move. The stretches focus on the areas where many people's bodies become inflexible, restricted and stuck. This is a good routine for people who can squat without pain (but it's fine if you can't get your heels flat on the floor) and want to experience a greater freedom and fluidity of movement.

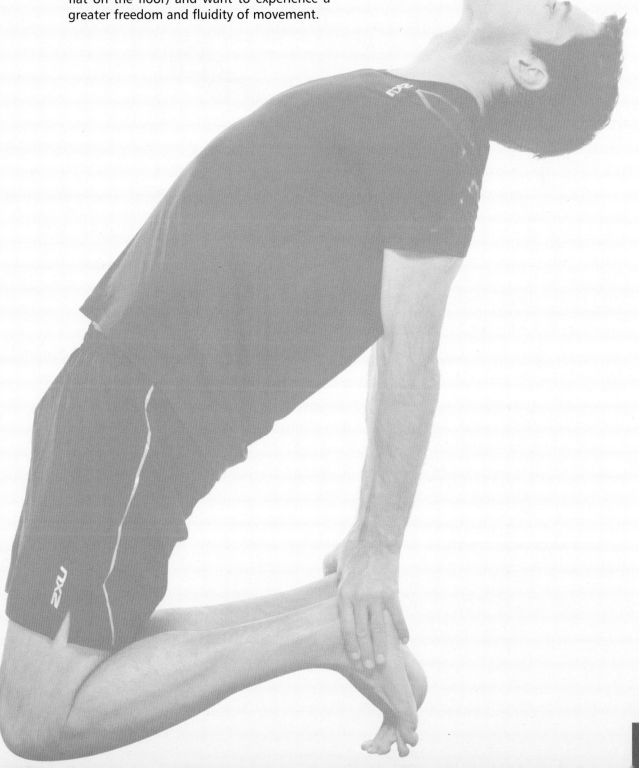

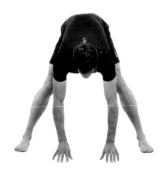

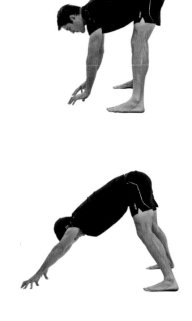

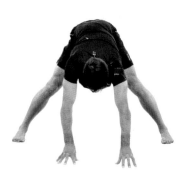

Main area and muscles stretched
Stretches the hamstrings.

Technique
Lean forward from your hips and while tensing the backs of your legs, walk your hands forward as far as you can comfortably go and then back toward and between your legs, again as far as you are comfortable. Walking forward and backward once is one rep.

Technique tips
Try also walking your hands around in a wide circle in front of you in one direction and then back in the other.

Suggested number of reps in one set
7–10.

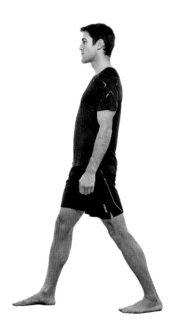
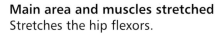
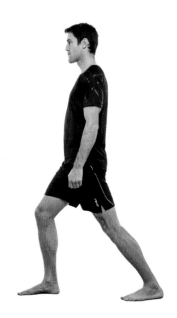

Main area and muscles stretched
Stretches the hip flexors.

Technique
Stand with one foot in front of the other and shoulder-width apart, with your hands on your hips. Tense the muscles on the front of your back hip as you lean forward, bending your knees to stretch your hip flexors.

Technique tips
Make the movement nice and smooth, without trying to go too far.

Suggested number of reps in one set
7–10 on each side.

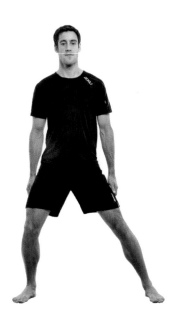 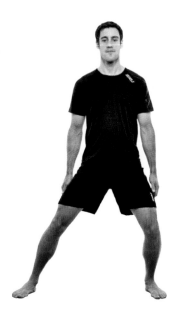 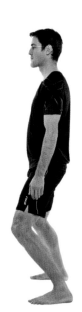

Main area and muscles stretched
Stretches the adductors.

Technique
Squat, with your tailbone tucked underneath you, pulling your feet together into the floor (they do not move, they just pull into the floor without rolling the knees inward).

Maintain that tension on the inside of the legs by squeezing the feet together and slide to one side to stretch the inside of the leg that is becoming straighter, be careful not to raise your hips, but slide evenly as if your bottom is moving along a shelf. Slide back all the way to the other side. Sliding to one side and then the other counts as one rep.

Technique tips
It can be hard to keep your hips tucked under if you are not used to it. Imagine that you are trying to flatten the curve in your lower back.

Suggested number of reps in one set
7–10.

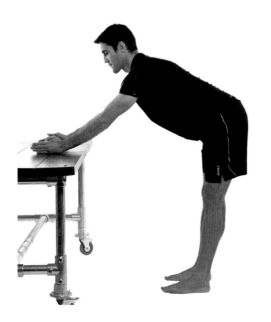
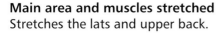
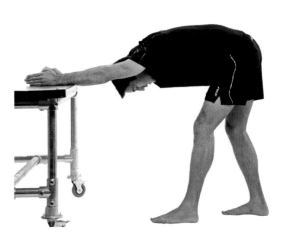

Main area and muscles stretched
Stretches the lats and upper back.

Technique
Put your hands down on a desk, parallel, on their sides, with your fingers facing away from you and facing each other, about one hand span apart.

Whilst continuously pulling your hands down into the desk, step back with one foot and lower your torso toward the floor, keeping your arms straight. Only go as far as you can comfortably go and then return easily to the starting position.

Technique tips
Make sure that you do not lean on your arms, but keep your weight on your supporting leg. It is fine to bend your knees.

Suggested number of reps in one set
7–10.

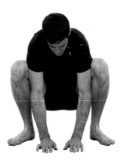
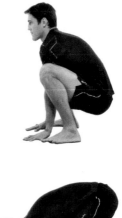
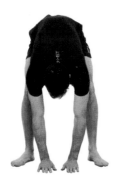
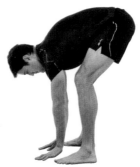

Main area and muscles stretched
Stretches the central hamstrings.

Technique
Sit in a deep squatting pose, tense the backs of your legs and then lift your bottom into the air, to stretch your hamstrings. As you push your bottom up, maintain the tension in the backs of your legs. Relax back down to the starting position and repeat.

Technique tips
Don't worry if your heels are not on the floor, or if you need to hold onto something sturdy to stabilize you.

Suggested number of reps in one set
7–10.

6. SQUATTING ADDUCTORS

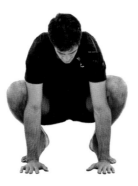 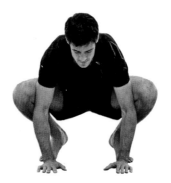

Main area and muscles stretched
Stretches the adductors.

Technique
Sit in a squatting position and place your arms between your legs. Lean forward and squeeze in with the legs, as your elbows simultaneously push the knees apart, to stretch your adductors.

Technique tips
The aim of this stretch is not to balance on your arms, only to lean forward to let gravity and your weight help to open your legs.

Suggested number of reps in one set
7–10.

7. QUAD STRETCH ON KNEES

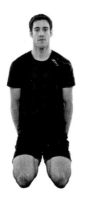 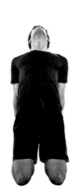 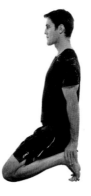

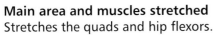 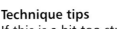

Main area and muscles stretched
Stretches the quads and hip flexors.

Technique
Kneel with your hands on your heels and sit on your heels with your shoulders pulled forward. Tense the front of your hips, and your chest as you sit up, pushing your hips forward and your shoulders back, always keeping your hands on your heels.

Technique tips
If this is a bit too strong, you can just do the kneeling quad stretch, where you can kneel up with your hands on your hips.

Suggested number of reps in one set
7–10.

Before

After

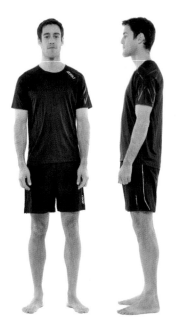 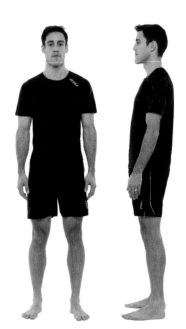

Brad is already very active and his training includes running, CrossFit, swimming, and other sports. He found that by incorporating the stretching into his life the hip pain he had been suffering from lessened, he got greater ranges of motion across all of the tests (between 0.4 and 7 inches) and after stretching every morning he felt that his mood and approach to the day were even more positive.

Brad's posture improved after a month of stretching, most noticeably in the openness of his chest (look at the space between his arms and torso at his waist), his hips became more open, and his head was less pushed forward. Changes such as these often have great effects on sports performance and I believe help people to avoid the deterioration in posture that is often associated with aging (but not a necessary part, from my point of view).

Hip Opener

This routine is designed to help open and free your hips, an area where many people, in the West especially, are tight and restricted. This has huge benefits as tension in the hips and pelvis can have a huge impact on the biomechanics of the whole body.

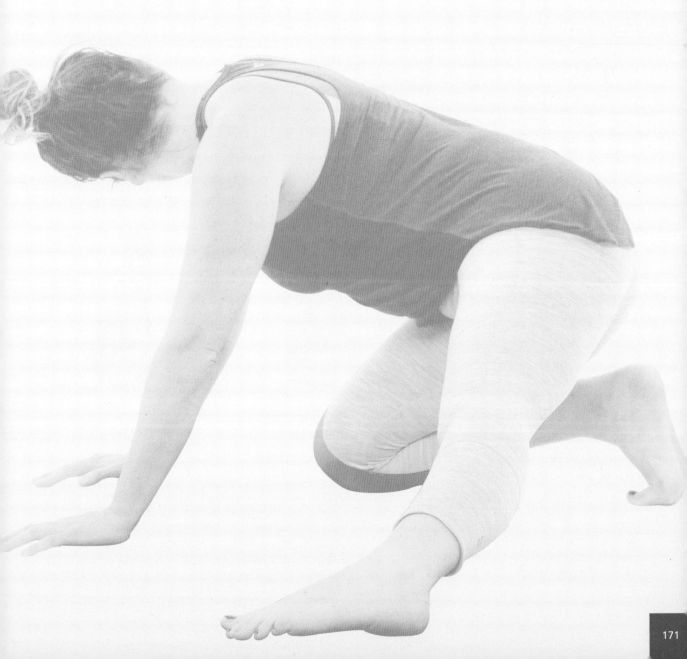

1. SITTING CROSS-LEGGED, LEAN FORWARD

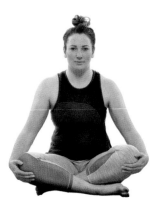
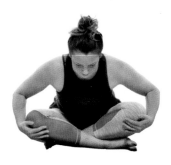

Main area and muscles stretched
Stretches the abductors.

Technique
Sit with your legs crossed and hands under your knees. Push your knees down into your hands continuously as you lean forward to stretch.

If you are naturally flexible and your feet go very close to your hips you will probably need to move them forward in order to get a stretch.

Technique tips
If you are very stiff then do not worry if your knees are very high. You can also move your feet further from your body if that is easier, and do not push too hard or lean forward further than is comfortable.

Suggested number of reps in one set
7–10.

2. SITTING WITH FEET TOUCHING

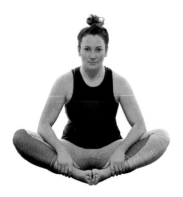
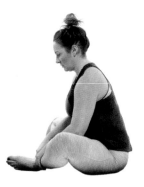

Main area and muscles stretched
Stretches the groin.

Technique
This is a strong stretch although it does not look like much from the outside! Sit with your feet together, holding your ankles and resting your arms on your legs. Push your legs up into your arms as your arms push against your legs and tip your pelvis forward to stretch your groin.

Technique tips
If this is hard to understand pretend that you have something in front of your hips and then try to push it forward with your hip bones. Try not to lean forward with your back, but concentrate on only shifting the hips forward. Pulling backward with your hands can also help you to rock your hips forward.

Suggested number of reps in one set
7–10.

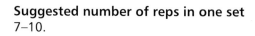

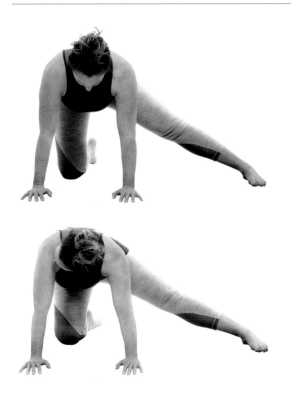

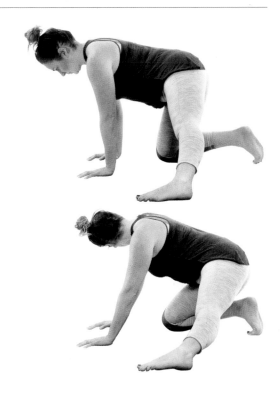

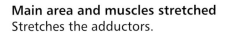

Main area and muscles stretched
Stretches the adductors.

Technique
On your hands and knees put one leg out to the side, straight and foot pointing forward. Continuously pull your foot down into the ground and slightly toward you as you sit back smoothly to stretch the adductors of your straight leg. And then return easily to the start position. Intensify the stretch by rolling your torso away from the leg you are stretching and looking away from your straight leg.

Technique tips
If your knee is sore on the floor, put some padding underneath it.

Suggested number of reps in one set
7–10 on each side.

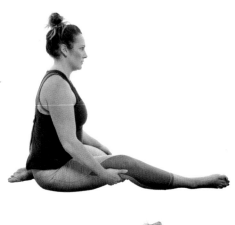
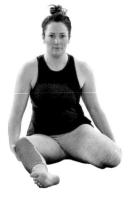
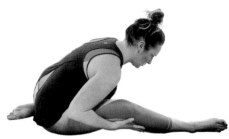
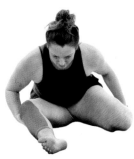
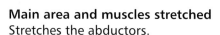

Main area and muscles stretched
Stretches the abductors.

Technique
Sit with your leg bent in front of you, with your knee at a greater than 90° angle. Support your knee with your hand or a block or cushion. The knee pushes down continuously into your hand as you lean forward to stretch the abductors and glutes. After leaning forward smoothly as far as you can comfortably go, return easily to the starting position.

Technique tips
Try not to bend your spine very much as you lean forward as this will not help your stretch.

Suggested number of reps in one set
7–10 on each side.

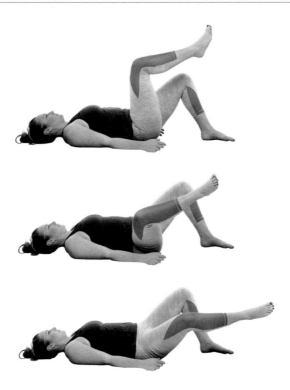

Main area and muscles stretched
Stretches the abductors.

Technique
Lie on your back and lift your leg up into the air with your knee bent at 90°. Tense all of the muscles in your hips as you slowly rotate your knee to the outside, down and out and then to the midline of your body, and up again in a circle.

Technique tips
Try to keep your hips flat on the floor and keep your abdominal muscles engaged so that you do not wobble from side to side. It may feel odd to tense your hips in this way; you can try thinking about trying to slow the movement down.

Suggested number of reps in one set
7–10 on each side.

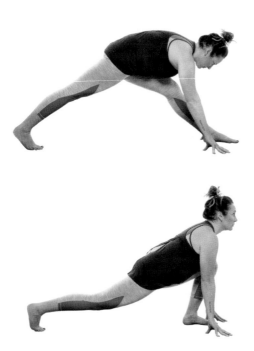

Main area and muscles stretched
Stretches the hip flexors and quads of the back leg.

Technique
Crouch as if you were getting into the starting position for a race, with both hands on the floor, and then push your back leg even further out behind you so that your legs are quite far apart. Push your bottom up into the air and tense the front of the leg which is behind you as your lower your hips down and lift your head as far as you can comfortably go, bending your front knee even more. Return easily to the start and repeat.

Technique tips
To generate even more resistance you can pull your back leg down into the ground and then move against that force. If this stretch is too difficult then you can kneel on one knee, pulling that knee forward as you lean forward, bending your front knee even more.

Suggested number of reps in one set
7–10 on each side.

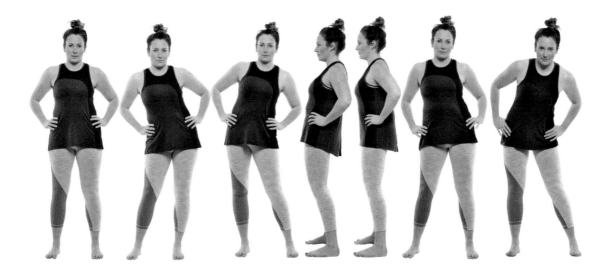

Main area and muscles stretched
Stretches the hips.

Technique
Stand with your feet hip-width apart. You are going to move your hips in eight directions out from the center point in the middle of your body, as if you were following the points of a compass. Before you move your hips, tense the muscles on the side of the body in the direction you are going. For example, before you push your hips straight out to the left, continuously tense the muscles on the outside of the left hip, as well as all of the muscles around your hips, upper thighs, back, and lower abdomen.

These are the directions you will stretch: to the left side, to the right side, forward, backward (do not sit back with your bottom, but keep your hips tucked under and push your tailbone backward), diagonally forward and left, diagonally backward and right, and then the reverse: diagonally forward and right, diagonally backward and left.

Technique tips
It can be hard to keep your tailbone tucked under if you are not used to it. You can think about it as trying to keep the small of your back as straight as possible.

Suggested number of reps in one set
5 in each direction in total.

Before

After

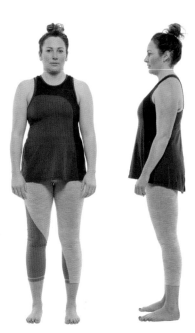

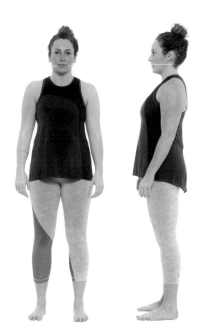

Carly is a sport rehabilitator and yoga and Pilates instructor. Through her month of stretching she experienced a marked reduction in hip and shoulder pain, had improved range of motion across almost all of the flexibility tests and also found it easier to do certain yoga poses that she has found more difficult in the past. In terms of health she found that she felt more energized and slept better.

Her posture improved a lot with her shoulders opening more, her head coming back, and her hips looking more open, as well as looking more toned all over. In addition to stretching she had also started taking supplements; aside from that there were no other variations in her exercise or diet.

In my practice I have seen people's postures improve from head to toe by working on freeing their hips.

Office Off

This routine was created for office workers and those who have to sit at a desk for long periods. All of the stretches can be done sitting on a chair at a desk and will only look slightly strange in the office! But they are well worth it, to help prevent hunching and tension from prolonged sitting.

If you do work in an office it would be beneficial to do at least one set of these once a day, but if you can do two sets, or one set twice a day, that would really help counteract the tightness and stiffness you can get from being immobile for hours.

Please bear in mind that you need a stable chair, not a chair with wheels or one that can tip over easily.

1. HIP FLEXOR AT CHAIR

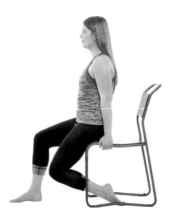 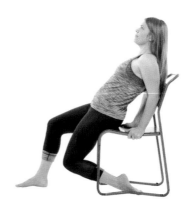

Main area and muscles stretched
Stretches the hip flexors.

Technique
Sit slightly at the edge of your chair, tuck your foot underneath the seat so your thigh is pointing down to the floor with your toes pointing backwards. Then, as you push your foot down into floor, lean back in one smooth, slow motion while holding the chair for stability. Come back to the starting position easily and gently and repeat.

Technique tips
It is better to have the top of your foot on the floor, but if this is sore, tuck your toes under your foot.

Suggested number of reps in one set
7–10 on each side.

2. HAMSTRING STRETCH AT CHAIR

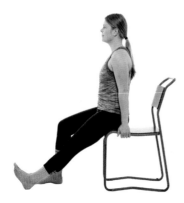 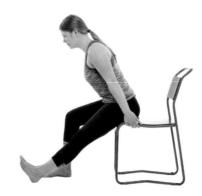

Main area and muscles stretched
Stretches the central hamstrings.

Technique
Sit with one leg out in front of you and your toes pointing toward your head. As your foot pulls itself down into the floor continuously to create tension, lean forward smoothly from your hips to stretch. When you have gone as far as you can comfortably go, return easily to the starting position.

Technique tips
Keep your toes pointing up throughout the stretch.

Suggested number of reps in one set
7–10 on each side.

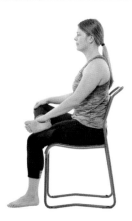
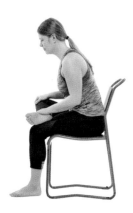

Main area and muscles stretched
Stretches the abductors.

Technique
Cross one leg over the other and that leg will push itself continuously down into your bottom leg. Smoothly lean forward as far as you can comfortably go, stretching the glute and outside of the upper leg, and then return to the upright starting position.

Technique tips
Only go as far as you can comfortably go and do not bend over from your back in order to go further, as it will not increase the stretch.

Suggested number of reps in one set
7–10 on each side.

4. ADDUCTOR STRETCH IN CHAIR

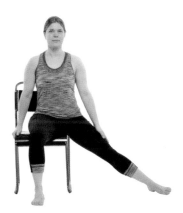
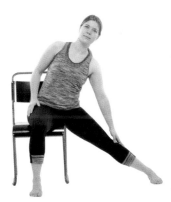

Main area and muscles stretched
Stretches the adductors.

Technique
Sit with one leg out to the side and straight. As the leg out to the side pulls down into the floor continuously, lean sideways toward that leg to stretch the adductors on that side.

Technique tips
You can put your hand on the straight leg, and slide it down as you stretch. This just helps to ensure you are stretching smoothly and evenly. You do not need to keep your foot flat on the floor if this is uncomfortable.

Suggested number of reps in one set
7–10 on each side.

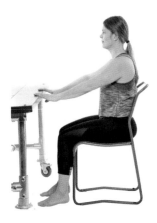 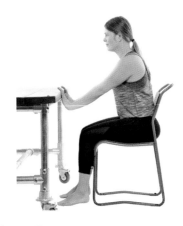

Main area and muscles stretched
Stretches your wrists and palms.

Technique
Rest your fingers on the edge of a desk and have your fingers and hands pushing down and into the desk. Lean forward with your body to push the heel of your palm down and forward, stretching your wrists and palms.

Technique tips
Only push as hard with your hands as you can without causing discomfort and always keep your elbows straight.

Suggested number of reps in one set
7–10.

6. CHEST STRETCH AT CHAIR

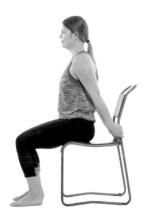 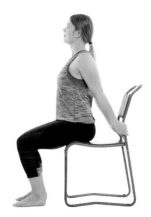

Main area and muscles stretched
Stretches the chest.

Technique
Hold the back of your chair and hunch your shoulders forward, tensing your chest and the front of your shoulders. Against that force push your torso forward to open and stretch your chest and shoulders as you pull against the chair with your hands.

Technique tips
As it is a small movement, the effectiveness of this stretch depends on a slightly higher level of resistance, which comes from tensing your chest muscles more, but only do this if it is comfortable.

Suggested number of reps in one set
7–10.

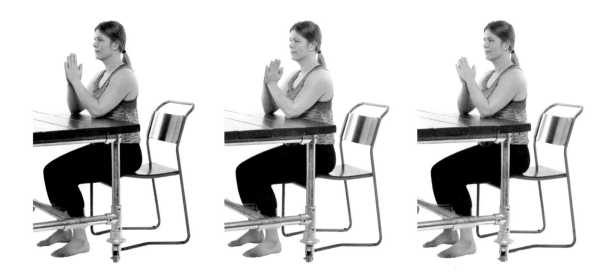

Main area and muscles stretched
Stretches the palms and fingers.

Technique
Put your hands together, with your elbows resting on the desk. Your hands resist each other as one pushes one way, and then the other pushes back. One wins and then the other. Only move from side to side.

Technique tips
You can have your fingers wide apart to change the stretch and you can also go as far to the side as you can reach comfortably.

Suggested number of reps in one set
7–10 on each side.

Before

After

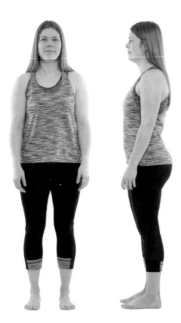

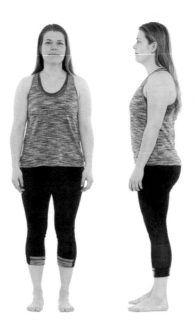

Daria is a nanny and keen allotment gardener, so she moves a lot throughout the day. She felt that the stretches opened her chest and also she felt more relaxed, energized and her back pain reduced. She had an improvement across all but one of the flexibility tests of 3–10 inches, which is a pretty spectacular benefit, especially for a routine that entirely takes place sitting down.

In terms of her posture, the stretching has brought her shoulders down and back, lessened the curve in her lower back and opened her hips, as well as creating more muscle definition. Her face also looks clearer and more toned.

Shoulder and Chest Opener

These stretches are great for improving posture, "unhunching" people, opening the chest and shoulders and helping to improve alignment in the upper body.

If you do hunch your shoulders, or experience neck or shoulder tension, this routine may work wonders for you. Please just be aware that if you are in any pain you should double check with a healthcare professional before starting to stretch, to make sure these stretches are appropriate for you.

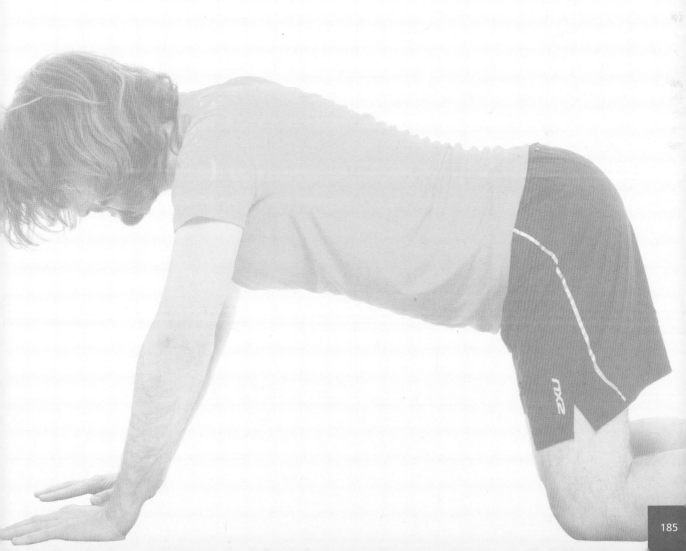

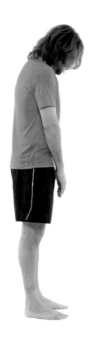 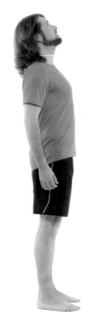

Main area and muscles stretched
Stretches the chest, front of the shoulders, and neck and the jaw.

Technique
This is a very simple stretch. Hunch your shoulders forward and look down. Then tighten your chest as you smoothly pull your shoulders back, lift your chin up, and push the sternum up and forward. Your hands will start facing inward and end up facing forward.

Technique tips
Create a stronger stretch by also tensing the front of your neck and the front of your shoulders as you lift your head and move your shoulders back against that force. Only add this in if you are not suffering from neck pain.

Suggested number of reps in one set
7–10.

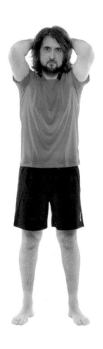
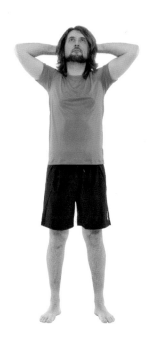

Main area and muscles stretched
Stretches the chest.

Technique
With your hands clasped behind your head and your elbows in front of you and close together, tense your chest continuously as you move your elbows back. Moving both elbows back once and returning easily to the beginning position is one rep.

Technique tips
Do not pull on your head with your hands or you may make your neck tense. Make the movement nice and smoothly. You do not need to look up as you stretch; but keep your head level.

Suggested number of reps in one set
7–10.

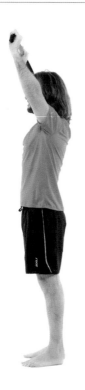
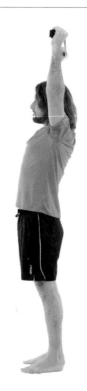

Main area and muscles stretched
Stretches the chest and shoulders.

Technique
Hold a yoga strap or a towel above your head, either wrapped around your hands or gripped firmly in both hands.

Let your hands face slightly outward, with your arms wide and your elbows straight. Start with your arms in front of your body (always high) and keep pulling your hands apart as you move your arms backward to stretch your chest.

Technique tips
If you get tired from having your arms above your head for so long it is fine to take a break mid-set. Also, if you are very flexible, only move your arms back as far as your shoulders stay in the same position in the joint—we do not want any contortionism in this stretch!

Suggested number of reps in one set
7–10.

4. CHILD'S POSE WITH RESISTANCE

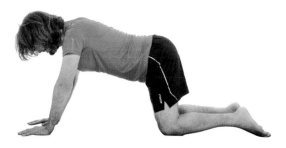 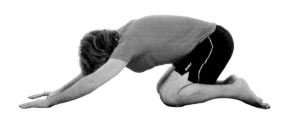

Main area and muscles stretched
Stretches the upper back, shoulders and upper arms.

Technique
On your hands and knees pull your hands down and back toward you into the floor. Keeping your elbows slightly bent and your back straight, smoothly sit back onto your heels.

Technique tips
Try to keep your back flat like a table and let your shoulders stay away from your ears as much as possible.

Suggested number of reps in one set
7–10.

5. PULLING ARM DOWN INTO FLOOR AND OPENING CHEST

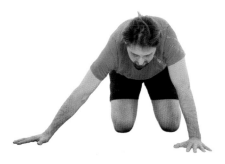 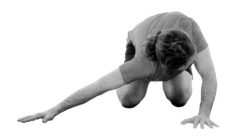

Main area and muscles stretched
Stretches the chest and inner arm.

Technique
On your hands and knees, put one arm straight out to the side, fingers pointing away from you. Pull it continuously down into the floor as you lower your upper body and twist your torso, looking away from your straight arm. Never stop pulling into the ground with the straight arm.

Technique tips
You can change the position of the arm out to the side by moving your hand a few inches forward each time. Bear in mind that in order to stretch effectively in this instance, you always need to sit back, away from your outstretched arm, wherever it is. This changes the area being stretched, giving you a more all-round stretch.

Suggested number of reps in one set
7–10 on each side.

6. CHEST STRETCH ON CHAIR

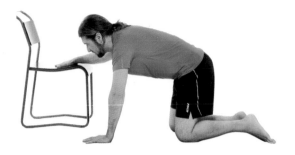 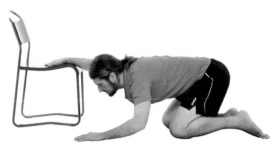

Main area and muscles stretched
Stretches the chest and inner arm.

Technique
Kneel with a chair in front of you and out to the side, one hand diagonally out, palm-down on the seat, pressing down continuously. Smoothly lean down to the floor to stretch your chest, by sitting back and bending your other arm.

Technique tips
If stretching with your arm straight hurts your elbow at all, just bend it slightly, and keep it at that position throughout the stretch.

Suggested number of reps in one set
7–10 on each side.

7. KNEELING PUSH-UP CHEST STRETCH

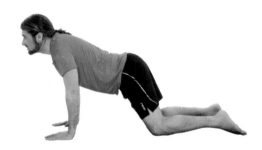 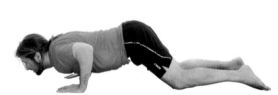

Main area and muscles stretched
Stretches the chest.

Technique
Get into a kneeling push-up with your hands wide and pointing slightly out, head facing up. Create tension in your chest then let your chest fall toward the floor in slow motion to stretch. Come up easily and quickly and repeat the stretch.

Technique tips
Visualize your shoulders becoming broader and your chest more open as you lower yourself down. If it is too hard to do 7–10 reps just start with 3–5 and build up.

Suggested number of reps in one set
7–10.

Before

After

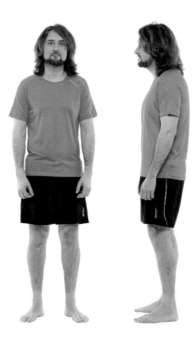

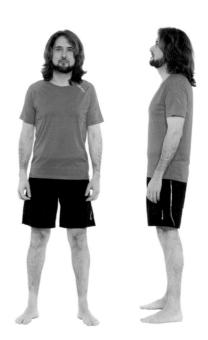

Javier is a guitarist so spends a lot of time bent over his guitar and in addition to that was in a motorbike accident a year ago and had persistent back pain that stopped him exercising. After stretching for a month his back pain had reduced so much that he could go to the gym again and exercise without pain. His flexibility measurements improved in almost all of the tests by 3–6 inches.

His posture has obviously improved, with his chest opening, shoulders coming back and his back straightening a lot. You can tell from the way Javier is standing that his balance looks much better, which is a common side-benefit of improving posture. Keeping up the stretching will help him to avoid hunching as he grows older and help to keep his back in good shape. He has also toned up overall, which is probably a combination of the stretching and his gym work.

Freeing the Legs

These leg stretches are great, both for people who work in an office and for people with sedentary lifestyles as the legs tend to get very tense when sitting all day. This routine also works well for "weekend warriors," helping to prepare the body for exercise and adventure after periods of inactivity. You can also use these stretches to keep the legs in good condition, which is especially important for those engaging in leg-dominant activities such as running and cycling.

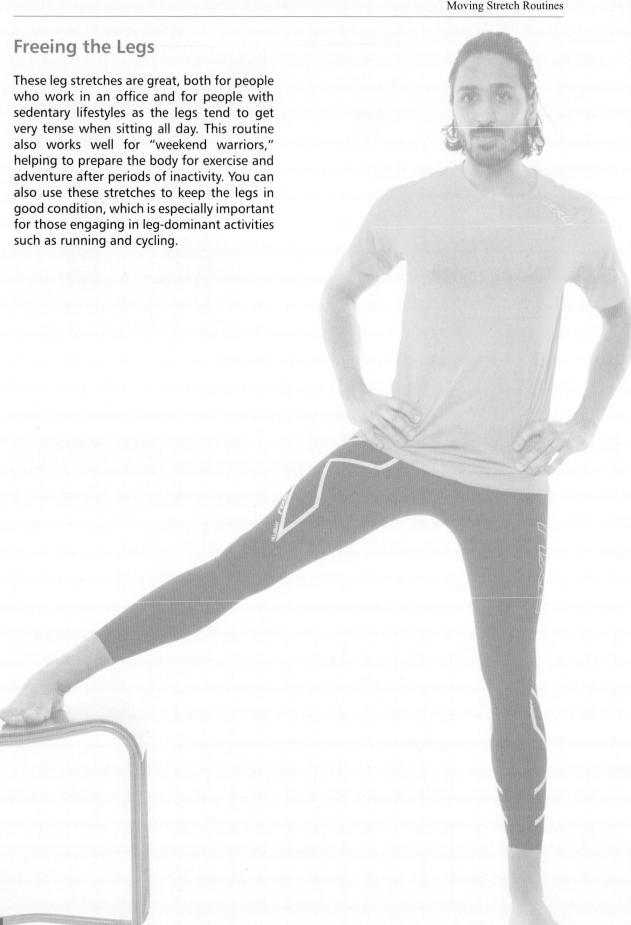

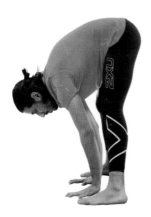
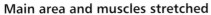
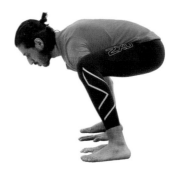

Main area and muscles stretched
Stretches the medial as well as central hamstrings.

Technique
Bend forward from the hips and tense your abdominal muscles to protect your back. If you can reach the floor, then touch the floor, but if not then hold your calves. Tense the inside/back of your thighs by pulling your feet in together and back, but without rolling the knees inward.

Squat gently down to a comfortable level and then push your bottom back up again, as far as you can comfortably, always tensing the inside back of your legs (medial hamstrings). One squat is one rep.

Technique tips
Do not worry if you cannot touch the floor or squat very low, just stay within a comfortable range and focus on moving against the resistance. The focus is on the quality of the movement against tension that you make, which should be smooth, comfortable, and consistent, rather than moving very far.

Suggested number of reps in one set
7–10.

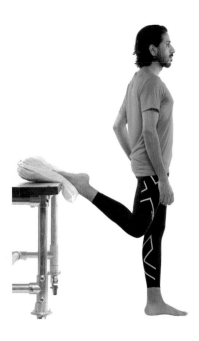 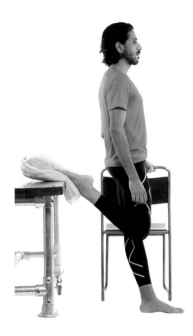

Main area and muscles stretched
Stretches the quads.

Technique
Rest your foot behind you on a table with a cushion on it or the back or side of a sofa. Push the foot of your bent leg back behind you (never downward) into the table or sofa continuously as you move your hips as far forward and then as far back toward your back foot as you can comfortably go, without pushing beyond any discomfort.

Hold onto something so that you are stable and keep your knee steady and straight as you stretch, do not let it wobble from side to side. Going forward and backward once counts as one rep.

Technique tips
Make sure that your standing leg is far enough away from the table so that you can move your hips forward as far as you can comfortably. If you are using a table then you can use a folded yoga mat, cushion, or pillow to protect your foot. Also make sure that when you move backward you do not "sit" at your hips, but keep your torso and the thigh you are stretching in one straight line.

Suggested number of reps in one set
7–10 on each side.

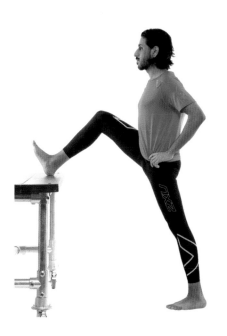 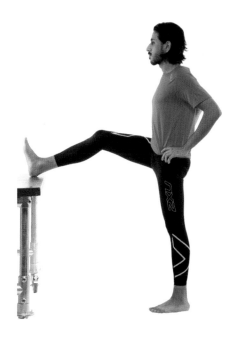

Main area and muscles stretched
Stretches the central hamstrings mainly.

Technique
Stand with one foot out in front of you on a table, step, or other secure surface. Bend the upper leg's knee as much as possible, and keeping the toes pointing upwards, continuously pull that foot down and back into the table. Now stretch by smoothly lengthening your leg by sticking your bottom out behind you.

Technique tips
Make sure that you start with your leg as bent as you can and engage your muscles and fascia by pulling your foot down and back right from the start, otherwise you will miss the opportunity to stretch through the whole range of motion. Do not put weight on your bent leg, only your standing leg. Only go as far back as you can comfortably go.

Suggested number of reps in one set
7–10 on each side.

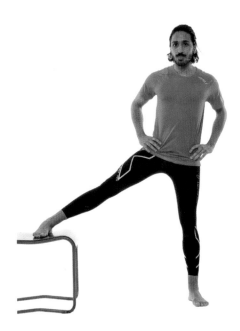
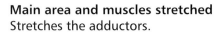
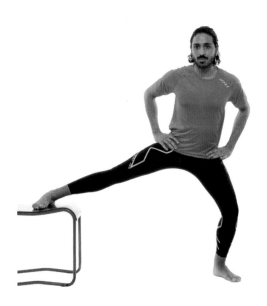

Main area and muscles stretched
Stretches the adductors.

Technique
With your foot up on a chair straight out to one side, keep that leg straight and pull the foot down into the chair continuously to engage the muscles of your inner thigh (adductors).

Keeping that force on, smoothly bend your standing leg as far as you can comfortably bend it to stretch your adductors and then return easily to the starting position. Bending and straightening the knee of your standing leg once counts as one rep.

Technique tips
Start with your standing leg straight and keep your weight on that leg. If you need to hold onto something to maintain your balance please do so. Make sure that you move smoothly and do not rush the movement. Also try not to bend forward from the hips as you bend your standing leg.

Suggested number of reps in one set
7–10 on each side.

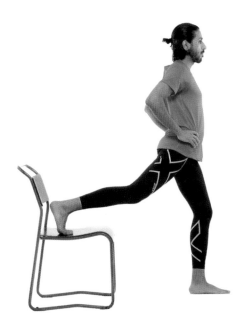
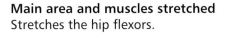
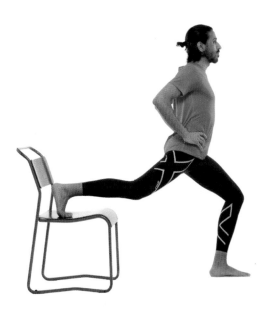

Main area and muscles stretched
Stretches the hip flexors.

Technique
Standing with your leg out behind you on a chair, step, or low wall, pull your back foot down and forward into the chair continuously to engage the muscles at the top and on the front of that thigh (the hip flexors). Smoothly and comfortably bend your standing leg to stretch the hip flexors of your back leg. Bending and straightening the knee of your standing leg once counts as one rep.

Technique tips
Try not to bend the back leg too much as you stretch, and try to stay as upright as you can throughout the whole stretch.

Suggested number of reps in one set
7–10 on each side.

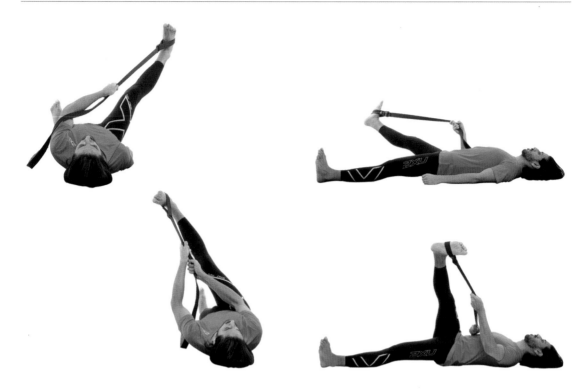

Main area and muscles stretched
Stretches the lateral hamstrings.

Technique
Stretch the outside/back of your thighs (lateral hamstrings) by lying down and putting the loop of a strap around one foot. Starting with the leg of that foot down and out to the side, keep it pulling itself in that direction as you pull it up and across your body, toward the opposite shoulder, with the yoga strap. The leg being pulled up and relaxing back down again once counts as one rep.

Technique tips
Try not to pull your leg down or toward your body with the strap, but up and across the body, so that you are pulling slightly higher than parallel to the floor, rather than down toward it. This helps to prevent us compressing the hip joint by accident. Keep the leg you are stretching straight throughout the movement and only go as far as you can comfortably go.

Suggested number of reps in one set
7–10 on each side.

Before

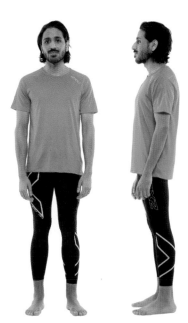

After

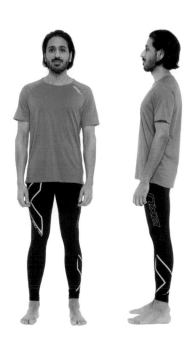

Avi did most of these stretches every day for 30 days alongside his normal Ashtanga yoga practice. As you can see from the before and after photos his alignment has improved and he is standing in a more natural and grounded way. The opening of his shoulders, broadening of his chest, the moving back to the midline of his head and reduction in hunching are all changes I see a lot in my regular clients and students, changes which I believe are a result of resistance stretching removing the restrictions in people's fascia which keep them in the wrong alignment.

Postural improvements like this often help people to be more confident as well as boost their performance in sports and yoga and help to reduce the chance of injury. It is interesting to see how stretching the legs has had a great benefit on the alignment of the upper body, showing just how interconnected the fascia and the whole body is.

Posture Perfect

These stretches are perfect for people wanting to generally improve their posture as it focuses on the tight areas that frequently pull people out of their naturally healthy alignment.

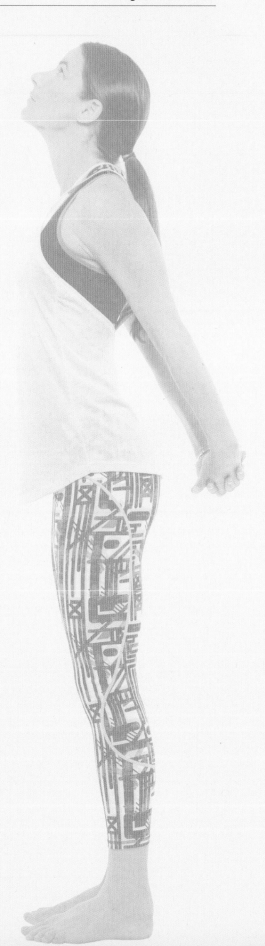

1. CHILD'S POSE WITH RESISTANCE

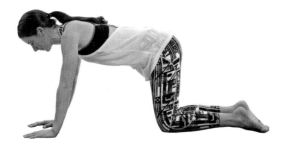 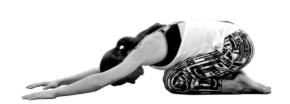

Main area and muscles stretched
Stretches the upper back and upper arms.

Technique
Get onto your hands and knees and keeping a slight bend in your elbows, pull back your hands down into the ground. As you continuously pull your hands down into the ground and back toward you, smoothly sit back on your heels.

Technique tips
If it is too easy then move your hands further forward and if it is too difficult, move your hands a little closer to your knees.

Suggested number of reps in one set
7–10.

2. HIP FLEXOR LOW LUNGE

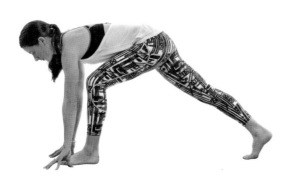 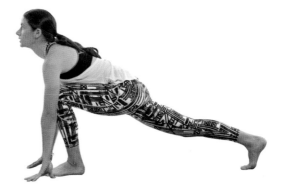

Main area and muscles stretched
Stretches the hip flexors.

Technique
Crouch as if you were getting into the starting position for a race, with both hands on the floor, and then push your back leg even further out behind you so that your legs are quite far apart. Push your bottom up into the air and tense the front of your hips as you lower your hips down and lift your head as far as you can comfortably go.

Technique tips
To generate even more resistance you can pull your back leg down into the ground from the very beginning of the stretch. You are stretching the front of the hip of the leg that is behind you.

Suggested number of reps in one set
7–10 on each side.

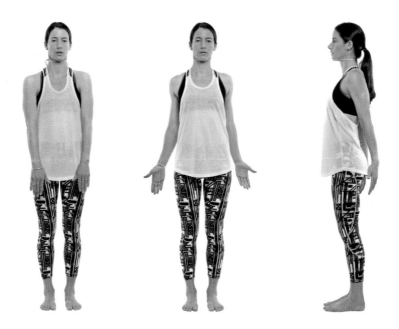

Main area and muscles stretched
Stretches the chest and the upper back.

Technique
In this stretch the arms rotate around you, with your palms always facing the body. Start with your arms straight down and in front of the body. Tensing your chest and shoulders, move your arms out to the sides and around behind you to stretch your chest.

Then tensing your back, move your arms back around to the front again, stretching your upper back. Keep your hands close to your body. Moving your arms backward and then forward counts as one rep.

Technique tips
This stretch is unusual in that you stretch in both directions, so it is really two stretches rolled into one. Because of this you have to remember to keep the resistance on in the correct area in order for the stretch to work. Try not to raise your shoulders.

Suggested number of reps in one set
7–10.

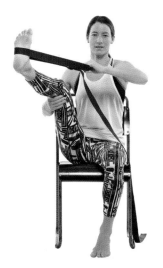 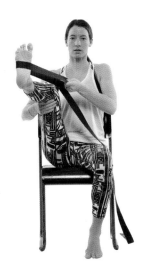 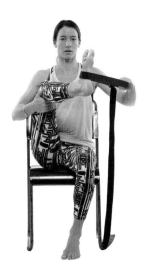

Main area and muscles stretched
Stretches the glutes.

Technique
Sit in a chair and make a loop with a yoga strap, belt or towel. Have one leg in the air, bent at 90°, with the hand of the same side holding the thigh under the knee to stabilize it. Place the loop around the foot and swing your foot outward as far as it can comfortably go. As you continue to pull your foot outward, smoothly pull your foot, with the yoga strap, across your body towards the opposite shoulder.

Technique tips
Please note that this stretch is all about pivoting, rather than the whole leg moving out to the side, therefore the thigh and knee stay in roughly the same place, while only the foot and upper leg move.

Suggested number of reps in one set
7–10 on each side.

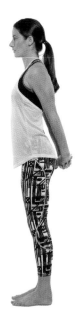 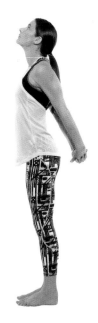

Main area and muscles stretched
Stretches the chest and the front of your shoulders.

Technique
Clasp your hands behind your back (or you can hold a yoga strap) with straight arms and hunch your shoulders forward. Tense your chest continuously as you lift your hands and open your chest.

Technique tips
To increase the area that is stretched, you can also tense the front of your neck and your upper chest and look upward at the same time as pulling your arms back.

Suggested number of reps in one set
7–10.

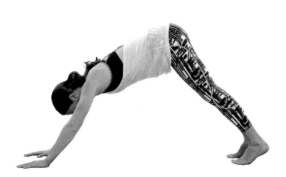 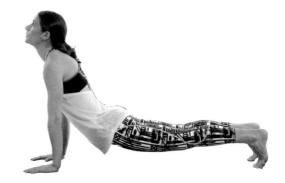

Main area and muscles stretched
Stretches the hip flexors.

Technique
Get into a full push-up position, and push your hips high up into the air. Tensing the front of your hips and abdomen, lower your hips toward the ground against that continuous tension, simultaneously looking up. Return easily to the starting position and repeat.

Technique tips
If this is too hard then you can do it in a kneeling push-up position, in which case you should let your feet point up into the air.

Please note that although it looks a bit like the yoga Cobra pose, it has a different effect as the stretch happens while you are moving and you keep the resistance on in the front of your thighs in order to ensure your hip flexors are being stretched. In addition do not let your thighs touch the ground and make sure you do not hold the pose, but keep moving through it.

Suggested number of reps in one set
5–7.

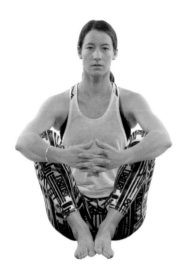
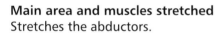
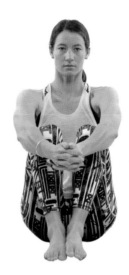

Main area and muscles stretched
Stretches the abductors.

Technique
Sit with your knees bent in front of your chest, feet together, arms around your legs and hands clasped (fingers interlinked). Start with your knees as far apart as they can go, and then as your knees push out continuously, straighten your arms and squeeze inward to stretch your abductors.

Technique tips
Try not to raise your shoulders as you do this, particularly if you have shoulder and neck tension.

Suggested number of reps in one set
7–10.

Before

After

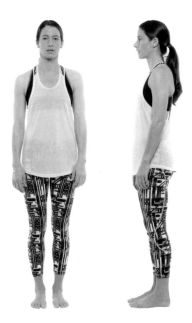
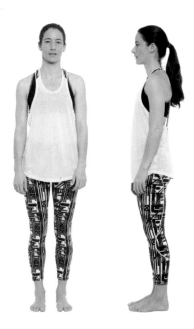

Nikki is a very experienced athlete (with the medals to prove it!) with a background in surf life saving. Although she competes at a competitive level she did not have a dedicated flexibility routine in place, so this project worked out well for her. Nikki's range of motion increased from 3 to 13 inches across all of the flexibility tests.

Her before and after photos show that her posture has not changed dramatically, as it was already very good. I would say that she looks more toned, her chest has opened a little and her neck seems a little longer. It is interesting that her posture could already be good and not needing to change very much, and yet she could have such dramatic improvements in her range of motion.

Stretchy Back

These stretches are designed to help free the back from tension and stiffness and through this create more movement in the rest of the body.

If you do suffer from back pain please consult a healthcare practitioner before starting to stretch and if you are fine to stretch, but do have back pain, then I suggest you ease into it and do fewer reps to start off with. Stretching the back can help you to boost your mobility as well as energy levels.

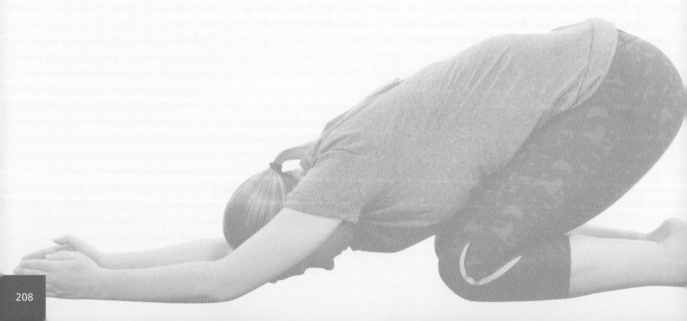

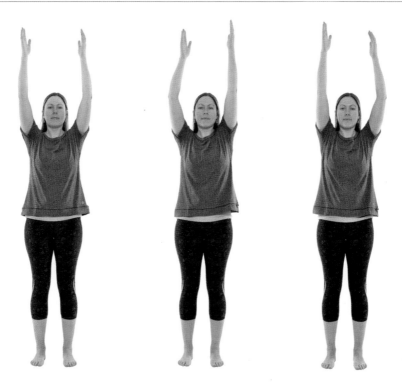

Main area and muscles stretched
Stretches the back and around the ribs.

Technique
Stand with your feet shoulder-width apart. Raise your hands out to the sides and up, and as you raise your hands imagine a line between them passing through the body.

As the line passes up through your muscles, tense each muscle that it passes through. With your hands above your head, parallel and facing each other, tense your back and the sides of your body and lift one hand up toward the sky, pushing as high as you can comfortably. Then easily return it to its natural position, keep the tension on in your muscles and push the other hand up toward the sky.

Technique tips
Make sure that your shoulders are as down and relaxed as they can be, except when being raised by the arm that is stretching. Try to be aware of your spine and ribs as you do this stretch and feel all of the muscles around them stretching.

Suggested number of reps in one set
7–10 on each side.

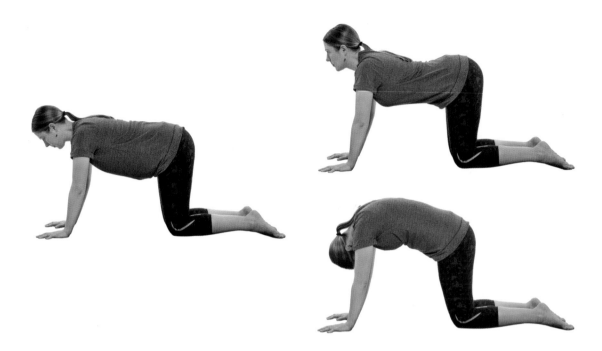

Main area and muscles stretched
Stretches the whole back.

Technique
Get onto your hands and knees and tense your back as you bend it down, lowering your belly button toward the floor. Keep the tension on as you arch your back up as far as you can go. From there you can push your back all the way down again and move fluidly from one to the other. Lowering and raising your back once counts as one rep.

Technique tips
Do not push through any pain and also remember to look up when your back is down, and down when your back is up.

Suggested number of reps in one set
7–10.

3. SIDE TO SIDE CAT

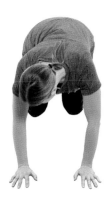 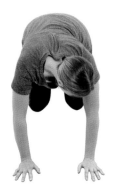

Main area and muscles stretched
Stretches the back and the sides of the torso.

Technique
Start in the same position as above but instead of going up and down you will be moving sideways. Tense your back and sides and move your head around to look down your left side, and curve your hips forward to the left toward your head. Come back to the starting position easily.

Technique tips
Try not to turn your head, but keep looking down so that your ear is moving closer to your hips rather than your chin.

Suggested number of reps in one set
7–10 on each side.

4. HIP FLEXOR PUSH-UP WITH WIDE LEGS

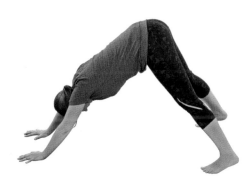 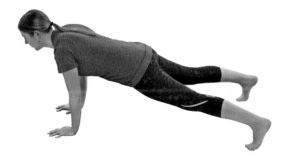

Main area and muscles stretched
Stretches the hip flexors.

Technique
Get into a full push-up position with your feet wide apart, and push your bottom high up into the air. Tensing the front of your hips and abdomen, lower your hips toward the ground against that continuous tension, as far as you can comfortably go.

Technique tips
Having the legs wide apart may be challenging, in which case you can have your feet closer together. The benefit of having the feet further apart is that it stretches a slightly different area. If you can do both, I suggest doing the one that feels the tightest.

Suggested number of reps in one set
5–7.

5. SITTING BACK ADDUCTORS

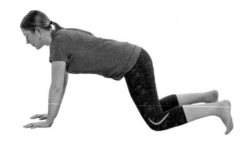 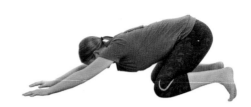

Main area and muscles stretched
Stretches the adductors.

Technique
On your hands and knees, place your knees even further apart and have your toes pointing outward as far as it is comfortable. Squeeze your knees into the floor and smoothly sit back. When you have gone as far as you can without discomfort, come back up to the starting position and repeat.

Technique tips
You may find that you need to move your hands a little further forward in order to get the full stretch.

Suggested number of reps in one set
7–10.

6. CHILD'S POSE WITH RESISTANCE

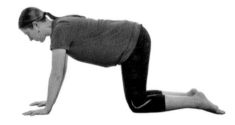 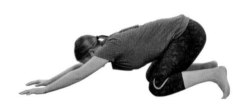

Main area and muscles stretched
Stretches the upper back, shoulders, and upper arms.

Technique
Still on your hands and knees, but with your knees back closer together (under your hips) pull your hands down and back toward you into the floor. Keeping your elbows slightly bent and your back straight, smoothly sit back onto your heels.

Do not stay at the end, but return up to the starting position easily and repeat.

Technique tips
As you can see in the picture you can either have your feet flat on the ground or toes tucked under, whichever suits you best. Try to keep your back flat like a table throughout the stretch.

You can experiment with how far forward or back to move your hands, to find the distance that gets you the best stretch.

Suggested number of reps in one set
7–10.

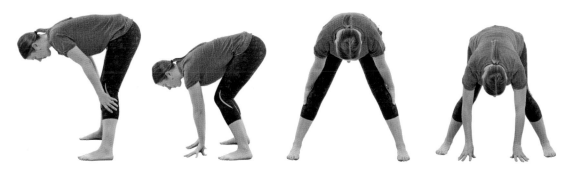

Main area and muscles stretched

Stretches the medial as well as central hamstrings.

Technique

Bend forward from the hips and tense your abdominal muscles to protect your back. If you can reach the floor, then touch the floor, but if not then hold your calves. Tense the inside/back of your thighs by pulling your feet in together and back, but without rolling the knees inward.

Squat gently down to a comfortable level and come back up again, always tensing the inside back of your legs (medial hamstrings). One squat (down and up again) is one rep.

Technique tips

Do not worry if you cannot touch the floor or go down very far, just stay within a comfortable range and focus on moving against the resistance. The focus is not on what your posture looks like during this movement, so much as the movement itself, which should be smooth, comfortable, and consistent.

Suggested number of reps in one set

7–10.

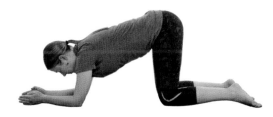
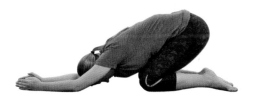

Main area and muscles stretched

Stretches the back and the lats especially.

Technique

On your hands and knees rest your elbows on the floor, underneath your shoulders and roll your arms onto their sides. Your palms should be facing each other and your forearms parallel. Pull your hands down and back toward you into the floor and smoothly sit back onto your heels.

Technique tips

Try to keep your back flat like a table and let your shoulders stay away from your ears as much as possible. To intensify the stretch move your hands further forward and to lessen the intensity move them closer to your knees.

Suggested number of reps in one set

7–10.

Before

After

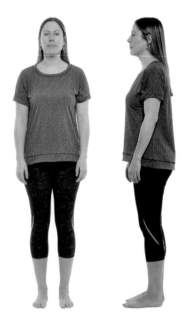
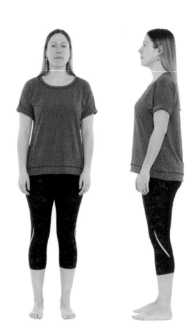

Milly is a teacher and training to be a yoga teacher. Like myself she classifies herself as "naturally inflexible" and before the stretching found that back pain was getting in the way of surfing, some yoga poses, and other daily activities. After only 2 weeks of stretching (due to getting a virus), her back pain had reduced a lot and she was sleeping better as a result. She also noticed marked improvements in her mood on the days that she stretched.

Milly's flexibility scores showed an improvement of 1–5 inches across all of the tests except for her left shoulder. Her posture improved with her head coming back and her shoulders opening. Her face also looks a bit brighter and more "open," and she looks stronger, which is a common result among my clients.

12 The Best Attitude for Stretching

> *"Don't keep reaching for the stars because you'll just look like an idiot stretching that way for no reason."*
>
> *Jimmy Fallon*

There is always a reason to stretch. When you start you may think that you are not doing it right, you may not have a specific issue that you need to resolve, you may think that 101 other things in your day are more important. Stretching holds amazing benefits for you that you will not experience unless you start. All you need to do is stretch at least a little bit every day or every other day, and be aware of how you feel, as well as open-minded about the results that you notice (which may not always be what you expect).

The truth is many people do not really like stretching and, generally speaking, inflexible people really, really do not like stretching. It is not that much fun to do something that you are quite bad at, and it can seem like the rewards just never show up. Even people who are generally quite flexible may not want to set aside time for a regular stretching practice, they may feel that it is not needed, that the direct benefits of stretching are unclear, or life just "gets in the way."

I feel that much of the unpopularity of stretching is down to how we have been taught to see it. It often feels like homework. So many clients tell me they know they "should stretch," probably in the same way they might tell a nutritionist they know they "should eat greens." If the word "should" doesn't dampen your enthusiasm, I don't know what will (which reminds me, I should be getting around to my tax return soon).

In fact, resistance stretching can be great fun and really enjoyable, engaging your muscles and fascia and stretching like an animal does make you feel very alive. My god-daughter, Maya, termed it "fighting stretching" (at only 5 years old she was already great at summing things up) and in a way it is, though not aggressive. You engage your muscles to pull one way and you push them another, fighting yourself. Fighting tension and weakness and lethargy. Waking yourself up and bringing yourself back to life. This is a good attitude to have when you stretch, so that you are present, engaged, and active.

It is important to know that stretching is not just something that you do "to" your body, as if your body were just a piece of machinery that needs servicing in order to work properly. There is much more to your body than just being a vehicle for your mind and emotions. The body has its own intelligence and needs and we need to be able to tap into that in order to be truly healthy. Often when we do not, we end up repeatedly becoming ill or injured and having to "fix" ourselves, because we did not listen to what our bodies had been telling us for minutes, days, months, or even years.

Bodies like it when you enjoy them, when you pay attention to them, play through them, move easily and in many different ways, breathe freely, drink enough water for them to stay clean internally and elastic, feel positive, challenge them enough that they stay "up-to-date," and appreciate them enough to take good care of them. They hate it when we stay in one position for hours and hours, eat without tasting our food, eat food that resembles flavored Styrofoam, drink too many alcoholic, sugary, or caffeinated drinks instead of drinks that hydrate us (because this adds toxins that make the body need even more water to flush them out) and they hate being forced to do things in the wrong way, especially when it harms them. This includes things such as stretching badly or having poor posture.

In terms of stretching, the body likes natural, healthy, satisfying, movements that build in intensity sustainably and indicate your desire for strength and a healthy range of motion. Often our goal-oriented minds approach the body with a "let's do this" attitude and we may try to use overly strong, rigid, or forced movements to push the body into greater ranges of motion, often before it is ready. The result of this approach is often stiffness, pain, and frustration as the body fails to play along. No wonder so many of us dislike stretching!

It is important to stretch in a way that not only gets your body on board, but makes your body feel more open, satisfied, strong, complete, and energized. This is not a "mind vs body = progress" scenario. This is a "mind + heart + technique + body = success" scenario. If you can embody this attitude and also pay attention to the points covered in this chapter, you should have a satisfying, sustainable, and transformative stretching practice in place in no time at all.

13 Motivation for Stretching

There is often a lot of unconscious resistance to making a change that either occurs immediately or sneaks up on us after the first flush of enthusiasm gives way to familiarity and a desire to spend more quality time with our sofas. Motivation is definitely my clients' biggest barrier to success with stretching, rather than the reasons I have been given over the years, including: lack of time, having a cold, lack of equipment, weather, clothing, other people being nearby, caring for children/pets. (Your children will love it when you to stretch, by the way, because you will probably feel happier and have more energy for taking them on walks, playing and affection! Pets also like to get involved; sometimes this is a bit of a hindrance but we can all learn from their enthusiasm.)

If you are a naturally motivated go-getting, alpha-stretching type you will probably not need this section and more than likely it will baffle you completely. On the other hand, if, like me, you have a strong lazy streak, it may be handy! And you can probably tell how lazy I am by the sheer diversity of ways to motivate you I have come up with. I hope one or two of these ideas will help to make stretching a permanent fixture of your life, rather than an infrequent afterthought. You may find that only one of these works for you. That's fine. Take whatever works and run with it.

1. Stretch to feel better, not to feel less bad

This is about attitude. If you are stretching to get over a particular ache or pain, then you will usually stop as soon as the pain goes away. This is not a recipe for long-term success. It is only through a long-term habit that we will see truly amazing results. When we keep in mind that we are getting a bit better each and every day we do our stretching, that we are working toward something, it is much easier to make time for our stretching and do it consistently, even when the duvet is soooo comfy and warm or when the sofa beckons.

2. Have a positive attitude around your stretching

Another attitude one! If you grimace and groan and call it "homework" you will probably be doing your stretching half-heartedly with poor technique and do less than you would otherwise. If you use your stretching session as time just for you, to get in touch with your body, relax, and maybe listen to some of your favorite music then you are much more likely to get into the zone and finish your session with a smile on your face, looking forward to the next stretch.

3. Be consistent, rather than a weekend warrior

It is better to do 10 minutes every day, or every other day, than 2 hours once a week. It takes the body time to transform because you are reprogramming it, and you need to send it consistent messages for how you want it to function. If you do want to do an extra long session that is great, just make sure you build up to it, so that the body can handle the changes you are asking it to make. If you try to jump ahead too fast the body will often respond by tensing more to protect you (against yourself!) and you may injure or strain yourself. Consistent habits create a solid foundation for success.

4. You are your habits

If you stretch for 10 minutes every day, your body will start to reflect that. Unfortunately it will also reflect how long you spend sitting, hunched over typing, or eating junk food. As well as your stretching it is important that you support the changes by eating food that helps the body to be healthy and strong, avoid hunching, staying immobile for long periods, and sitting for longer than necessary. The good news is that usually when we start to stretch we become attracted to healthier habits. I suggest you listen to these impulses and let the stretching positively influence other areas of your life.

5. You can stretch almost anywhere

I stretch on public transport, at home, in cafes, in parks, in short almost anywhere I feel like it. I take other people into account and I am considerate but there are many stretches that are convenient to do almost anywhere. For example, you can stretch your glutes almost wherever you are sitting, whether on a park bench or on public transport, by sitting with one leg across the other, and leaning forward gently. Or you can stretch your arms on a tree in the park, stretch your adductors while you do the washing up, by squatting slightly, tensing your inner thighs and moving from side to side. Of course you have to put safety first and only do it if it is practical, but if you are time poor, then slotting stretches in here and there where you can may be the way forward. Just make sure you do not stretch too hard before you are warmed up as if you are stopping and starting your body will be "cold" every time you start again.

6. Set a regular time to stretch

This one is great for people who work well with set routines. You can set a stretching alarm on your phone, stretch as soon as you get up, schedule your session in your calendar, set a regular time with a friend, or stretch during a specific regular TV show. I think that stretching without distraction is often best, but at the end of the day, if you are doing it then you are ahead (even if you do need TV, music, or a live orchestra accompanying you to motivate you)!

7. Stretching pays dividends

Aside from the reward of feeling much better and healthier, if you are a rewards-motivated person, then setting rewards for specific stretching goals can really work. For example, if you stretch every day for 7 days you go and do something you enjoy with a friend. If you stretch 6 days a week for 4 weeks then you buy yourself something you've been wanting or go and do something you've wanted to do for a long time. They do not have to cost money, they just have to motivate you personally. And it is rewarding to work toward something and have the satisfaction of having completed each milestone.

8. Not stretching is missing out

If you are the opposite of a rewards-motivated person and are more motivated by trying to avoid pain then you can always set yourself a task that you like less than stretching that you have to do each time you miss out on a stretching session you had committed to. It could be 50 press-ups, it could be cleaning the toilet, eating Brussels sprouts, or putting money in a pot (you could give it to charity). Whatever *does not* float your boat. As long as it is safe, ethical, and healthy you can give it a shot. (I'd much rather go after the rewards personally!)

9. Stretching likes company

Sometimes there is nothing like other people to motivate you. Why not gather a few friends at your house or a local park to stretch together, and then there is always the option of a cup of tea and a catch up after as a reward! You can do group stretching in lots of ways; 10 minutes at the end of your running/cycling/rowing/ultimate Frisbee session with friends, meet up in the park with friends/local Mums/local Dads or Mums and Dads, as a warm-down from your regular dance class, family stretch time, and more. Why not think of a way that suits your lifestyle? Even if it culminates with a drink in the pub with your friends, at least your day featured some good stretching as well!

10. As a regular add-on

I am realistic and I know that many of my clients are parents and/or have full-on jobs. If you are in this category, then it may suit you to do your stretching as an add-on to your regular workouts, Pilates sessions, daily walk or run, or any other specific times that you exercise. This is a good way to stretch because you are in the mood to do something physical, you will find it easier to remember to do it, and it does not take up too much extra time. If this is the way that works for you, that is great. Please try and make sure you do at least 10 minutes and really focus on your stretching to get the most out of it.

> *"Satisfaction lies in the effort, not in the attainment. Full effort is full victory."*
>
> *Mahatma Gandhi*

Find Your Reason to Stretch

Finally, if you are still having real problems "finding the time" to stretch (i.e., you don't really want to do it) I have also found that connecting to your most relevant personal goal is the best way to motivate yourself. Why not see if one of these is true for you and it will help you to stick to stretching for long enough to see real results:

- I want to feel and look younger and slow ageing as much as possible.
- I want my body to move responsively and easily.
- I want to have great posture.
- I want to avoid injury so I do not miss out on playing my sport or other physical activity.
- I want to improve in, and excel at, my sport.
- I want to stay fit and strong enough to run around with my future kids/grandkids.
- I do not want to put up with this pain any longer.
- I do not want to put up with this tension any longer.
- I want to have strong and healthy muscles and bones.
- I want to improve my biomechanics.
- I do not like being so tight and limited.
- I do not like hunching over.
- I want to stop feeling so tired and demotivated.
- I want to look and feel confident and energetic.
- I want to feel energized and have a spring in my step.
- I want to be able to move gracefully without restriction.
- I want to become the best I can be physically.

Although a many of these goals also require effort outside of stretching (such as specific training to improve in your sport), stretching may contribute a lot toward it. So what is the goal you are you really trying to achieve? Many of my clients say they want to be more flexible in general, but 99% of the time there is a much more personal and individual reason underlying this, such as "I am tired of feeling less than 100%," or "I am sick of bending down like an old man," or "I want to swim faster and better."

> *"And the day came when the risk it took to remain tight inside the bud was more painful than the risk it took to blossom."*

Anaïs Nin

Many things can be improved through improving your physical state, including health, mood, energy levels, mental clarity and even success. Think about what really matters to you and see if stretching can help you with that goal. Even if it cannot help directly, being fit and healthy, tall and open is an advantage pretty much all of the time. By finding your unique reason to stretch you will be able to work toward it with focus and enthusiasm for what you are about to achieve.

When You are Feeling Pretty Rubbish and DO NOT Want to Stretch

Here is a bit of extra motivation for those who cannot think of anything worse than stretching right now. Your body, your mind, your emotions all take their cue from you. You set the tone. If you are feeling a bit rubbish it can be hard to take that first step. We have all been there. If you are feeling very low on energy, low on motivation or resistant to making an effort or a change, just accept that—do not fight it. Just start with one stretch every day if you need to. Accept that part of you will not want to put the effort in, not want to change, or not want to feel better. If you have felt this way for quite a long time, then your personality will have adapted to feeling this way and seeing the world in the way that matches your state. Change can be scary for parts of you that have grown used to your current state. Do not fight those feelings, just thank them for their input and coax them with encouragement and smiles,

or maybe just ignore them while you start to stretch!

If you do one stretch when you'd rather do anything else, then you should feel really good about it, because that initial step can be harder than a 10 mile run, Ironman, or 3 hour stretching session is for someone who loves to move. Getting through the initial avoidance, resistance, suspicion, or outright hatred of change starts with one tiny step. This tiny step is then followed by lots of tiny steps and then a few medium steps, repeated medium steps, and then a big step. This is how people accomplish great things. But for right now, if getting out of bed 5 minutes early to do one stretch is what you can do, do that. And give yourself a big "well done!!"

The more you stretch, the more you feel like stretching and the easier it is to fit it in, because you always find space for things you like to do. So there really are no excuses, you will be able to fit this into your life, and you can choose to start today.

Normally I do not like the classic scare tactics used in marketing, but it can help people to understand the consequences of their choices. So here we go … If you are still not yet sufficiently motivated to get up and stretch, just picture something for me: yourself in 10 years. Yet rather than the old "nothing has changed" scenario, imagine that your stiffness is much stiffer, your pain worse, your hunch more hunched, and you look and feel older, maybe your face is a little greyer. Now picture yourself in 10 years having stretched regularly: more youthful, with great posture and color in your cheeks, quite possibly a sparkle in your eye. Which version of yourself will you choose? Moving Stretch® is definitely not the only way to stay youthful and healthy, but since you already have this book …

> *"Do it now. Sometimes 'later' becomes 'never'."*

Anonymous

References

Appleton, B.D. (2010). Stretching and flexibility: everything you never wanted to know. [Online]. Retrieved from: http://www.bradapp.com/docs/rec/stretching/ (accessed: April 18, 2016).

Avison, J.S. (2015). *Yoga: Fascia, Anatomy and Movement*. Edinburgh: Handspring Publishing.

Baker, J. (2016). Telephone interview. May 16, 2016.

Battié, M.C., Levalahti, E., Videman, T., Burton, K., and Kaprio, J. (2008). Heritability of lumbar flexibility and the role of disc degeneration and body weight. *Journal of Applied Physiology, 104*(2), 379–385.

Berrueta, L. Muskaj, I., Olenich, S., et al. (2015). Stretching impacts inflammation resolution in connective tissue. *Journal of Cellular Physiology, 231*(7), 1621–1627.

Bowman, K. (2014). *Move Your DNA*. Chichester: Lotus Publishing.

Brinol, P., Petty, R.E., and Wagner, B. (2009). Body posture effects on self-evaluation: a self-validation approach. *European Journal of Social Psychology, 39*(6), 1053–1064.

Coulter, D.H. (2010). *Anatomy of Hatha Yoga: A Manual for Students, Teachers, and Practitioners*, Marlboro: Body and Breath.

Cristopoliski, F., Barela, J.A., Leite, N., Fowler, N.E., and Rodacki, A.L. (2009). Stretching exercise program improves gait in the elderly. *Gerontology, 55*(6), 614–620. [Online]. Retrieved from: http://www.ncbi.nlm.nih.gov/pubmed/19713691 (accessed: April 11, 2016).

Day, C.S., Moreland, M.S., Floyd Jr, S.S., and Huard, J. (1997). Limb lengthening promotes muscle growth. *Journal of Orthopaedic Research, 15*: 227–234.

Dolan, A.L., Hart, D.J., Doyle, D.V., Grahame, R., and Spector, T.D. (2002). The relationship of joint hypermobility, bone mineral density, and osteoarthritis in the general population: the Chingford Study. *Journal of Rheumatology, 30*: 799–803.

Freudenrich, C.C. (2001). *How Ultrasound Works*. [Online]. Retrieved from: http://www.physics.utoronto.ca/~jharlow/teaching/phy138_0708/lec04/ultrasoundx.htm (accessed: May 3, 2016).

Fritz, S. (2013). *Sports and Exercise Massage*, 2nd edn. Missouri: Elsevier.

Guimberteau, J.-C. A pioneer in looking at fascia in living bodies, there are some very interesting videos on Professor Guimberteau's webpage. Retrieved from: http://www.guimberteau-jc-md.com/en/videos.php (accessed: September 29, 2016).

Harper, D. (2016). *Online Etymology Dictionary*. Retrieved from: http://www.etymonline.com/index.php?term=fascia (accessed: February 19, 2016).

Hedayatpour, N., and Falla, D. (2015). Physiological and neural adaptations to eccentric exercise: mechanisms and considerations for training. *BioMed Research International, 2015*, 1–7. [Online]. Retrieved from: http://www.hindawi.com/journals/bmri/2015/193741/ (accessed: April 18, 2016).

Hedley, Gil (n.d.) *Fascia and Stretching: The Fuzz Speech*. [Video]. [A funny, interesting, and endearing view of fascia]. Retrieved from: https://www.youtube.com/watch?v=_FtSP-tkSug (accessed September 29, 2016).

Hurley, J. (2012). "Barefoot" Clark stays one step ahead. *The Telegraph,* April 24, 2012. [Online]. Retrieved from: http://www.telegraph.co.uk/finance/businessclub/9221917/Barefoot-Clark-stays-one-step-ahead.html (accessed: May 5, 2016).

Ingber, D. E. (2003). Tensegrity I. Cell Structure and Hierarchical Systems Biology. *Journal of Cell Science.* 116, 1157–1173. [online]. Retrieved from: jcs.biologists.org/content/116/7/1157 (accessed: November 25, 2016).

Katzmarzyk, P.T., Gledhill, N., Pérusse, L., and Bouchard, C. (2001). Familial aggregation of 7-year changes in musculoskeletal fitness. *Journal of Gerontology: Biological Sciences, 56A*(12), 497–502.

Kim, J.H., Jung, E.S., Kim, C.H., Youn, H., and Kim, H.R. (2014). Genetic associations of body composition, flexibility and injury risk with ACE, ACTN3 and COL5A1 polymorphisms in Korean ballerinas. *Journal of Exercise, Nutrition and Biochemistry, 18*(2), 205–214.

Kjaer, M. (2015). Stress loading and matrix remodeling in tendon and skeletal muscle: cellular mechano-stimulation and tissue remodeling. In: Schleip, R., and Baker, A. (eds), *Fascia in Sport and Movement.* Edinburgh: Handspring Publishing, pp. 39–43.

Klingler, W. (2015). Physiology and biochemistry. In: Schleip, R., and Baker, A. (eds), *Fascia in Sport and Movement*. Edinburgh: Handspring Publishing, pp. 21–29.

Kokonnen, J., Nelson, A.G., Eldredge, C., and Winchester, J.B. (2007). Chronic static stretching improves exercise performance. *Medicine and Science in Sports and Exercise, 39*(10), 1825–1831.

Langevin, H.M. (2013). *The Science of Stretch*. Retrieved from: http://www.the-scientist.com/?articles.view/articleNo/35301/title/The-Science-of-Stretch/ (accessed: May 16, 2016).

Lazier, E.L. (1943). *Anatomy of the Dogfish*. Redwood City: Stanford University Press.

Lederman, E. (2015). Human movement performance. In: Schleip, R., and Baker, A., (eds). *Fascia in Sport and Movement.* Edinburgh: Handspring Publishing, pp. 83–91.

Levin, S.M. (2013). Biotensegrity, the mechanics of fascia. In: Schlep, R., Findley, T.W., Chaitow, L., and Huijing, P. (eds). *Fascia: The Tensional Network of the Human Body.* London: Churchill Livingstone, pp. 137–142.

Marek, S.M., Cramer, J.T., Fincher, A.L., et al. (2005). Acute effects of static and proprioceptive neuromuscular facilitation stretching on muscle strength and power output. *Journal of Athletic Training, 40*(2), 94–103.

McDougall, C. (2015). *Natural Born Heroes: The Lost Secrets of Strength and Endurance*. London: Profile Books.

Minshull, C., Eston, R., Bailey, A., Rees, D., and Gleeson, N. (2014). The differential effects of PNF versus passive stretch conditioning on neuromuscular performance. *European Journal of Sport Science, 14*(3), 233–241.

Muscolino, J.E. (2012). *Fascial Structure*. Illinois: American Massage Therapy Association.

Myers, T.W. (2012). *Are You Aging or Just Drying Out?* Retrieved from: https://www.youtube.com/watch?v=wL1ZVarr1R8 (accessed: May 25, 2016).

Myers, T.W. (2014). *Anatomy Trains: Myofascial Meridians for Manual and Movement Therapists*, 3rd edn. Edinburgh: Churchill Livingston/Elsevier.

Myers, T.W. (2016). Skype interview. April 25, 2016.

O'Sullivan, K., McAuliffe, S., DeBurca, N. (2012). The effects of eccentric training on lower limb flexibility: a systematic review. *British Journal of Sports Medicine, 46*(12), 838–845. [Online]. Retrieved from: http://bjsm.bmj.com/content/46/12/838.long (accessed: April 18, 2016).

Oschman, J.L. (2009). The development of the living matrix concept and its significance for health and healing. [Online]. Retrieved from: http://bti.edu/pdfs/Oschman_Living-Matrix-Concept.pdf (accessed: May 16, 2016).

Oschman, J.L. (2015). *Energy Medicine: The Scientific Basis*, 2nd edn., London: Churchill Livingstone.

Paoletti, S. (2006). *The Fasciae: Anatomy, Dysfunction and Treatment*. Seattle, WA: Eastland Press, pp. 151–161.

Peper, E., and Lin, I.M. (2012). Increase or decrease depression: how body postures influence your energy level. *Biofeedback, 40*(3), 125–130.

Pipelzadeh, M.H., and Naylor, I.L. (1998). The in vitro enhancement of rat myofibroblast contractility by alterations to the pH of the physiological solution. *European Journal of Pharmacology, 357*(2–3), 257–259. [Online]. Retrieved from: http://www.sciencedirect.com/science/article/pii/S0014299998005883 (accessed: May 15, 2016).

Porcari, J., Bryant, C.X., and Comana, F. (2015). *Exercise Physiology (Foundations of Exercise Science)*. Philadelphia: F.A. Davis.

Reynolds, G. (2014). *The First 20 Minutes: The Surprising Science of How We Can Exercise Better, Train Smarter and Live Longer*. London: Icon Books.

Rodriguez, M.R. (2015). Understanding mechano-adaptation of fascial tissues: application to sports medicine. In: Schleip, R., and Baker, A. (eds). *Fascia in Sport and Movement.* Edinburgh: Handspring Publishing, pp. 185–193.

Schleip, R. (2003). Fascial plasticity—a new neurobiological explanation. *Journal of Bodywork and Movement Therapies, 7*(1), 11–19. [Online]. Retrieved from: http://www.fasciaresearch. com/images/PDF/InnervationExcerpt.pdf (accessed: May 8, 2016).

Schleip R., Klingler W., and Lehmann-Horn, F. (2005). Active fascial contractility: fascia may be able to contract in a smooth muscle-like manner and thereby influence musculoskeletal dynamics. *Medical Hypotheses, 65*(2), 273–277. [Online]. Retrieved from: http://intl.elsevierhealth.com/ journals/mehy (accessed: February 22, 2016).

Schleip, R., Jager, H., and Klingler, W. (2012). What is "fascia"? A review of different nomenclatures. *Journal of Bodywork and Movement Therapies, 16*, 496–502. [Online]. Retrieved from: http:// fasciaresearch.de/Schleip2012_FasciaNomenclatures.pdf (accessed: May 17, 2016).

Sherman, A.J., Cherkin, D.C., Wellman, R.D., et al. (2011). A randomized trial comparing yoga, stretching, and a self-care book for chronic low back pain. *JAMA Internal Medicine, 171*(22), 2019–2026. [Online]. Retrieved from: http://archinte.jamanetwork.com/data/Journals/ INTEMED/22535/ioi15070_2019_2026.pdf (accessed: April 4, 2016).

Silvers, H.J., and Mandelbaum, B.R. (2007). Prevention of anterior cruciate ligament injury in the female athlete. *British Journal of Sports Medicine, 41*(1), 52–59. [Online]. Retrieved from: http:// www.ncbi.nlm.nih.gov/pmc/articles/PMC2465242/ (accessed: May 17, 2016).

Slauterbeck, J.R., Fuzie, S.F., Smith, M.P., et al. (2002). The menstrual cycle, sex hormones, and anterior cruciate ligament injury. *Journal of Athletic Training, 37*(3), 275–278.

Starrett, K. (2015). *Becoming a Supple Leopard*, 2nd edn. Las Vegas: Victory Belt Publishing.

Steckl, C. (2014). How the three pillars of exercise benefit mental health. Retrieved from: https:// www.mentalhelp.net/blogs/how-the-three-pillars-of-exercise-benefit-mental-health/ (accessed: May 4, 2016).

Vorman, J., Worlitschek, M., Goedecke, T., and Silver, B. (2001). Supplementation with alkaline minerals reduces symptoms in patients with chronic low back pain. *Journal of Trace Elements in Medicine and Biology, 15*(2–3), 179–183.

Walker, B. (2011). *The Anatomy of Stretching*, 2nd edn. Chichester: Lotus Publishing.

Wojtys, E.M., Huston, L.J., Lindenfeld, T.N., Hewett, T.E., and Greenfield, M.L. (1998). Association between the menstrual cycle and anterior cruciate ligament injuries in female athletes. *American Journal of Sports Medicine, 26*(5), 614–619.

Woodyard, C. (2011). Exploring the therapeutic effects of yoga and its ability to increase quality of life. *International Journal of Yoga, 4*(2), 49–54.

Worrell, T.W., Smith, T.L., and Winegardner, J. (1994). Effect of hamstring stretching on hamstring muscle performance. *Journal of Orthopaedic and Sports Physical Therapy, 20*, 154–159.

Yamamoto, K. Kawano, H., Gando, Y., et al (2009). Poor trunk flexibility is associated with arterial stiffening. *American Journal of Physiology, 297*(4), 1314–1318. [Online]. Retrieved from: http:// ajpheart.physiology.org/content/297/4/H1314.long (accessed: February 23, 2016).

Zorn, A. (2007). Physical thoughts about structure: the elasticity of fascia. *Structural Integration, March 2007*, 15–17. [Online]. Retrieved from: http://www.somatics.de/ZornElasticity.pdf (accessed: September 30, 2016).

Further Resources

If you want to know even more about Moving Stretch, stretching or fascia, here is a selection of great sources of information.

Moving Stretch
movingstretch.com
Online videos and resources for stretching.

Go to movingstretch.com/iboughtthebook for free extras.
Share your success story with us on twitter @moving_stretch or on our Facebook page @movingstretch.

Anatomy Trains
anatomytrains.com
Tom Myers' system of Anatomy Trains is a wonderful view of the anatomy of fascia and there are interesting blog articles too!

Functional Fascia
functionalfascia.com
Julian Baker's educational dissection courses give an amazing insight into anatomy for bodyworkers and movement specialists.

Gil Hedley's Fuzz Talk
youtube.com/watch?v=_FtSP-tkSug
A funny, interesting and endearing view of fascia.

Fascial Fitness
fascialfitnesstoday.com
This is a collaboration between Dr Robert Schleip and Tom Myers and offers strategies for training the fascia.

Buckminster Fuller On Tensegrity
youtube.com/watch?v=7JwOX4PlO2A
In this youtube video, Fuller describes tensegral structures in his own words.

Fascia Research Society
fasciaresearchsociety.org
A great resource for fascia research and events

The Anatomy of Stretching: Your Illustrated Guide to Flexibility and Injury Rehabilitation (Brad Walker)
This is a great book for those who would like more information on the anatomy of the muscles they are stretching, with fantastic illustrations.

Dr Jean-Claude Guimberteau
guimberteau-jc-md.com/en/videos.php
A pioneer in looking at fascia in living bodies, there are some very interesting videos on his webpage.

There are many more resources out there, but these are some of my favorites to recommend to beginners.